P9-CQQ-952

Brush Your Teeth!*

*and other simple ways to stay young and healthy

David S. Ostreicher, DDS, MS, MPH

To my loyal staff, my lovely wife, Brenda, and my beautiful brilliant daughters, Skye and Brie.
Thank you for giving me so much to look forward to.

Brush Your Teeth! and other simple ways to stay young and healthy

Copyright © 2009 David Ostreicher. All rights reserved. No part of this book may be reproduced or retransmitted in any form or by any means without the written permission of the publisher.

Published by Wheatmark®
610 East Delano Street, Suite 104
Tucson, Arizona 85705 U.S.A.
www.wheatmark.com

International Standard Book Number: 978-1-60494-095-4 (paperback)
International Standard Book Number: 978-1-60494-115-9 (hardcover)
Library of Congress Control Number: 2008922374

Contents

If Things Are So Bad, How Come We're Living Longer?

Follow along with me for a moment. Practically everything you read or see on television tells you that pollution is everywhere; our food supply is full of dangerous germs, unhealthy additives, and hormones; we eat too many foods with trans fats; there's an obesity epidemic; and nobody is exercising. We're fat and we're lazy. We watch too much TV; we're getting bombarded by UV rays through holes in the stratosphere; we're at risk from AIDS, SARS, mad cow disease, and bird flu.

This is all true.

But at the same time, we're living longer. How come the average life expectancy in the United States today for a man is 77 years, while a hundred years ago it was just 47?[1] The same is true for women. A hundred years ago, a woman could expect to live only to 50; today, she can expect to live to 80. And a hundred years ago, nearly 10 percent of children died in infancy; today the infant mortality rate is 0.7 percent.[2]

If our food is worse, if pollution is worse, if there's less ozone and more radiation—if everything is worse, why are we living so much longer?

The answer is simple. It's *hygiene*. We're cleaner. We have a cleaner water supply, better sewer systems, and yes, better personal hygiene.

This is not to say that the medical advances of the last 50 years haven't been spectacular. They have been. Clearly, antibiotics, vaccines, medicines, and surgical techniques have saved countless lives. But don't underestimate the magic of good sanitation.

Chances are you're going to live a long time. (Well, a long time based on human standards of the past millennium. If you're old enough to read, and relatively healthy at the moment, you've got a great chance of living past 80. However, inasmuch as the universe is more than 12 billion years old, you're just a tick of the universe clock. But don't let that depress you.) Getting back to reality, we know what will probably get you. Most people in the western world will die of either heart disease or cancer. That's the way it is. Sorry. And that's the way it's been for more than 50 years.

That isn't necessarily bad news. Not that you're likely to die of these things—that *is* bad news. But you can *do* something to keep any of those things from happening too soon. The good news is that heart attacks are largely preventable! More good news: many cancers are largely preventable. So, the bottom line is that the two major causes of death in the United States are largely preventable. And prevention isn't particularly hard to do. In fact, it's so simple.

Just 50 years ago, four of the top ten causes of death were infectious diseases. These infectious diseases were—and still are—linked to poor sanitation. These include diseases of infancy; influenza and pneumonia; tuberculosis; and nephritis (kidney infection).[3] One mechanism of studying these deaths is the death rate. Fifty years ago, the death rate for these combined illnesses was 110.7.[4] That means that out of every 100,000 Americans in 1950, 110.7 people died as a direct result of an infectious disease. (I know that number is a little strange, since there's no such thing as 0.7 of a person. Although we all know some people who act like they "aren't all there!")

Today, only pneumonia, influenza, and nephritis are still on the top ten list.[5] The death rate from these killers has gone way down. The combined death rate for infectious diseases is 43.7—considerably less than half that of earlier years. Most public health professionals would agree that the dramatic decrease in these deaths is due to improved sanitation. Better living conditions. Cleaner environments. Better hygiene.

But it doesn't end there. The number-one killer of them all, heart disease, also has had a significant decline in the past 50 years. The age-adjusted death rate in 1950 for diseases of the heart was 586.8. In 2003, the age-adjusted death rate for diseases of the heart was only 232.3. How did that happen? Certainly, better medical care, better medicines, and early diagnosis all played a role. But there's one more possible reason: better hygiene.

During the past 20 years, there has been increasing evidence that heart disease may be, at least in part, the result of inflammation caused by a bacterial infection of the arteries.[6, 7, 8] And guess where the bacteria comes from: your mouth and your gums!

So that's it. Your mother was right! The first step to health is to wash your hands and face, and brush your teeth. It's *far* more important than you think.

By keeping your hands clean, you help break the chain of transmission for dangerous microbes. By brushing your teeth, you help prevent periodontal disease, which is directly linked not only to heart disease, but also to other serious health problems, such as diabetes and premature birth.[9, 10]

Both of these simple, commonsense steps take little time and cost practically nothing. You don't need any special equipment beyond a bar of soap and a toothbrush, and you don't need any special training. It's almost hard to believe that something so easy could have such an impact on your health. Trust me. It's true.

So if just washing your hands and brushing your teeth can have such an impact, what about other simple health measures, like eating right, reducing your stress level, getting enough sleep, exercising regularly, and wearing your seatbelt? Your common sense tells you that these are sensible steps that work. Sensible as they are, we often find them hard to do. We lead busy lives, and we can't always eat right or get enough exercise. As for getting enough sleep and reducing our stress levels, those are goals that often seem totally out of reach.

Even though many of us weigh too much, exercise too little, and are kept up at night by worries, we focus too much on small things. For instance, we decide that eating only organic food will somehow magically make us healthier. We forget that too many organic cookies are just as fattening as too many regular old cookies—and a lot more expensive.

But let's say you decide to stick with organic cookies. That's great—you're probably helping the environment in some tiny way. But are you helping your health? Yes, but only if you also take these steps:

- Wash your hands when you get back from the store.
- Brush your teeth after eating the cookies.
- Eat the cookies in moderation as part of an overall good diet.
- Get a good nights' sleep after having a late-night cookie snack.
- Lower your stress level (eating isn't the healthiest way to do that).
- Exercise to work off the calories from the cookies.
- Wear your seat belt driving to and from the cookie store.

Any one of these steps will do a lot more to keep you healthy than eating organic cookies will. Put them all into action, and you'll be doing more for your health than you would by eating organic *everything*.

Putting It into Perspective

Let's keep things in perspective. Yes, it's possible that you might get bird flu, or West Nile virus, or some other scary disease, but it's actually pretty unlikely. In the meantime, you might be neglecting the sensible health precaution of keeping your vaccinations up to date. Since the introduction a few years ago of a vaccine for hepatitis A, cases are down nearly 90 percent.[11] You're a lot more likely to be exposed to hepatitis A than to West Nile virus—especially if you work with children or in health care—and it's a disease that can now be easily and painlessly

(OK, it's a shot, so *almost* painlessly) prevented. So, have you been vaccinated for it? No?

Heart disease is the leading cause of death among Americans.[12] We worry about it—for good reason—and try to fend it off by popping pills for high cholesterol and high blood pressure. Do the pills work? Yes, because they lower those magic numbers. No, because they don't deal with the underlying problems that make you need the pills in the first place. And even while people take the pills, they complain about the costs and the side effects. There are simpler, tried-and-true ways to improve your heart health: don't smoke; maintain a healthy body weight; drink alcohol in moderation; eat a high-fiber, low-fat diet; and exercise regularly. Small improvements in lifestyle can have big payoffs in health. It's just common sense. It's so simple.

The same thing applies to other health worries. We spend so much time obsessing over our cholesterol numbers and other health issues that we forget about the fifth leading overall cause of death: accidents. The death rate from accidents has been rising alarmingly. In fact, accidents are the leading cause of death for people between the ages of one and forty-one. A major cause of accidental deaths is car crashes, but the death rate for these actually has been dropping in recent years. The same is true for deaths from workplace accidents. Nowadays, the most likely place for a fatal accident—or a serious injury—turns out to be your own home. Your odds of being shot at the office by a disgruntled employee are much lower than your odds of being hurt or killed by an accidental fall at home.[13] But which scenario keeps you up at night? Here's my suggestion: instead of worrying about shooting sprees, take some common sense precautions to prevent home accidents. You might start by putting an inexpensive, nonslip mat into the bathtub.

It's So Simple

I've been a dentist for nearly 30 years. I've also got a master's degree in public health and another master's degree in biology and nutrition. After years of treating patients and teaching nutrition and health to graduate students, I've learned a lot about the realities of living a healthy life. I know that what we teach and what people actually do are two very different things. One big reason for the difference is that what we teach tends to be way too complex.

In this book, I hope to simplify things for you. I want to explain how small, simple, inexpensive steps can lead to big improvements in your health and well-being. Just washing your hands more often is a good example. Make handwashing a habit, and chances are you won't get sick as often with colds and other illnesses. The same is true for just about everything else I discuss in this book. Brush your teeth more often, eat better, sleep more, exercise regularly, reduce your stress, and avoid accidents, and you'll feel better both physically and mentally. And, chances are you'll live better and longer.

Of course, all that is easy to say and harder to do. But not a lot harder, as this book shows. As you read through the chapters, you'll see how simple it all really is. You don't have to make huge changes in your lifestyle—small steps work much better. As you'll learn, living a better, healthier life really just takes something you already have in abundance. That's right: your common sense. And it's so simple!

CHAPTER 1

Brush Your Teeth!

Even if I wasn't a dentist, and even if I hadn't been explaining it to my patients for the last 30 years, I'd still be saying this: Brush your teeth.

That's a pretty basic message, and you've probably already gotten it, in the sense that you probably do brush your teeth at least once a day. You probably think you're doing it to keep your teeth clean and reduce the risk of cavities. You are, but you're also doing something else that's just as important. When you brush regularly, you're helping to prevent periodontal or gum disease. That's important in and of itself, because gum disease is the main cause of tooth loss. By keeping your gums healthy, you're helping to keep your smile healthy, too. But just as important is the fact that periodontal disease is a risk factor for some serious health issues. These include heart disease, stroke, diabetes, respiratory problems, osteoporosis (a condition in which bones become thin and brittle), and premature birth. By preventing gum disease, you're also going a long way toward preventing the problems linked to it. And it's quite likely that, if you do have gum disease, treating it can improve your overall health.

Your Early Warning System

We dentists like to say that your mouth is your early warning system for your health. If you have gum disease or other dental problems, there's a good chance that you're on the way to other health problems—or may even have them already.

Let's start by defining exactly what I mean when I say "dental problems," beginning with your teeth. Of all the parts of your body, your teeth are the dumbest. Why? Because other parts of your body can heal themselves if something goes wrong. Break a bone, for instance, and with proper medical treatment, it will heal. Cut your skin—same thing. Get sick with a cold, and your body fights off the infection. But if you get a cavity, the tooth can't heal itself. In fact, your teeth are so dumb that the only thing that happens if you get a cavity is that it gets worse, not better, over time. And when you go to a dentist to have a cavity treated, the only thing the dentist can do is stop the problem at that point. I can fill your cavity, but your tooth will never heal itself and return to what it was before the decay set in.

Obviously, your teeth are an important part of your mouth, and you want to keep them not only healthy, but attractive. Brushing them regularly is the single most important thing you can do for your teeth. Brushing cleans not only your teeth, but also—and equally important— the area along the gum line. It stimulates your gums and is crucial for preventing both cavities and periodontal disease.

Second in importance to brushing your teeth is flossing them. Flossing removes the bits of food and other debris between your teeth where your toothbrush can't reach.

If you don't brush your teeth regularly, tooth decay and gum disease are sure to follow.

Periodontal Disease Defined

If you've just learned that you have periodontal disease, you might not be too happy, but at least you're not alone. About 80 percent of all adult Americans have some form of periodontal disease.[14] In many cases— and I hope in yours—it's diagnosed in the early stages of mild gum inflammation and can easily be treated. If not, it's possible that the soft tissue and bones that hold your teeth have been damaged; in the worst cases, you could end up losing teeth. Fortunately, today's treatments mean that we can often stop gum disease before it gets to the more severe stages.

Being told they have gum disease often comes as a big surprise to my patients.

"But I brush my teeth every day," they protest, "and I don't have any other dental problems. Sure, my gums bleed a little when I brush. But that's not serious, is it?"

"What?" I respond with amazement. "If your hands bled every time you washed them, you sure would think *that's* serious, wouldn't you?"

Sadly, brushing alone isn't usually enough to prevent periodontal disease, and even people who have never had a cavity can get it. To understand why, let's take a closer look at what happens in your mouth.

Your mouth, my mouth, everyone's mouth is full of bacteria. Around the clock, those bacteria combine with the saliva in your mouth to form a sticky, clear, microscopically thin film that coats your teeth. That film is called plaque, and it's the culprit behind both tooth decay and gum disease.

When you brush your teeth, you remove the plaque—if you brush long enough and correctly. Flossing removes more plaque from the spaces between your teeth. (I'll talk more about the best ways to brush and floss later in this chapter.) Even the most dedicated brushers and flossers, however, can't get all the plaque off. Most of us aren't all that dedicated—we tend to skimp on and rush through our dental hygiene. The end result: the plaque that isn't removed hardens up and forms tartar. (The technical term is "calculus." But that gets confused with the math class my kids take in high school: calculus. Both are very hard! So let's stick with the old term, "tartar.") There are two big problems with tartar: it's a great place for bacteria to hide out and breed, and you can't remove it yourself. The only way to get the tartar off your teeth is to have a professional cleaning by a dentist or dental hygienist.

If all that plaque and tartar stays on your teeth, the bacteria can really go to town. On your teeth, the bacteria feed on sugars in your diet and breed merrily away. As a byproduct of digesting the sugar you give them, the bacteria excrete acid. Now, one microscopic bacterium producing acid isn't going to do much damage, but many millions of them will. All that acid erodes the extremely hard enamel that covers your teeth. Eventually—and this could take as long as several years—the erosion wears all the way through the enamel. Now you have a cavity in the tooth. You know it because the tooth may ache and be sensitive to cold or heat. If you don't get to a dentist to get the cavity treated, it gets worse. The cavity reaches the soft inner pulp of your tooth, causing an infection called pulpitis. The pulp swells, but because it's within the hard tooth, there's no place for the swelling to go. The swelling presses on the blood vessels that nourish the tooth, cutting off the blood supply, and the tooth eventually dies. In the meantime, of course, you're experiencing extreme pain.

If the infection spreads beyond the pulp of the tooth and into the root, you get an abscess, which is even more painful. And if the infection spreads into your jaw and the surrounding tissue, it's more painful yet. Finally, the infection can enter your bloodstream and cause a body-wide infection that can be very serious, even life threatening.

OK, so cavities are bad. You probably already know that, because chances are you've had a few. You might even have had a cavity that got into the root and needed the special (and painful and expensive) treatment known as a root canal. What you may not know is that cavities aren't the leading cause of tooth loss. Gum disease is.[15]

Gum disease begins in much the same way that cavities do. There's a shallow trough where your gums meet your teeth. Just as leaves can clog up a gutter, plaque and tarter can build up in this trough. Bacteria love it—they get in there, breed away, and give off toxins.

Your body's response to those toxins is just like its response to toxins anywhere: it revs up your immune system and sends infection-fighting cells to the area. In the process of fighting off the bacteria, those cells release enzymes. Unfortunately, the enzymes have a nasty side effect. They break down gum tissue.

The infection caused by the bacteria, and your body's response to it, makes your gums swell, redden, and bleed easily. If the infection is mild, it's called gingivitis. Treating gingivitis is fairly easy and painless. All you really need to do is brush and floss more often and more thoroughly, use an antimicrobial mouthwash, and have your teeth cleaned regularly. Gingivitis can almost always be reversed without any long-term damage to your teeth and gums.

Ignore the gingivitis, however, and the infection will get worse, and the damage to your gum tissue will become more severe. Avoid treating gingivitis long enough, and it will turn into periodontitis. Now you've really got a problem—a painful, time-consuming, and expensive problem.

Periodontitis literally means "infection around the tooth." In a healthy mouth, your gums are nice and firm; they fit tightly around the base of your teeth, forming a sort of seal that protects the roots of your teeth. If you have periodontitis, your gum tissue breaks down badly. It pulls away from your teeth and forms little "pockets" that contain infection. You officially have periodontitis instead of gingivitis when the infection reaches the tooth socket.

Periodontitis can happen to just one tooth or a lot of teeth, or even to all of them. As with gingivitis, your body's immune system tries to fight off the infection as the plaque spreads below the gum line. What happens then isn't pretty. The toxins given off by the bacteria, along with the enzymes and other substances your body makes to fight off the bacteria, start to break down the connective tissue and bone that hold your teeth in place. Eventually, if you don't seek treatment, the breakdown is so severe that the teeth loosen and may even have to be removed.

Long before that happens, you've been getting warning signs (not counting what your dentist has been telling you). These are some common symptoms of periodontal disease:

- Bad breath that won't go away
- Red and/or swollen gums
- Bleeding or tender gums
- Sensitive teeth
- Painful chewing

Some people are more susceptible than others to gum disease. If you have any of these risk factors, you're more likely to develop it:

- Smoking. The biggest and most avoidable risk factor of all is smoking. If you smoke, periodontal disease is another outstanding reason to quit.
- Hormonal changes. This one applies only to women. The hormonal changes that come with menstruation, pregnancy, and menopause can lead to greater risk.
- Diabetes. People who have diabetes are at greater risk of infection everywhere, including their gums. (I'll talk more about diabetes later in this chapter.)
- Medications. Many medications can impact oral health and affect dental treatment. Hundreds of common medications—including steroids, cold remedies, antihistamines, diuretics, painkillers, high blood pressure medications, and antidepressants—can cause side effects such as dry mouth and gingival overgrowth. These medications also can change the type of bacteria living in your mouth, allowing disease-causing varieties to flourish.
- Caffeine and alcohol. Both of these can cause dry mouth. This condition leaves the mouth without enough saliva to wash away food and neutralize plaque and bacteria. The net effect is to make you more susceptible to periodontal disease.
- Stress. If you're under a lot of stress, your body is less able to fight off infections, including periodontitis. This is such an important issue that I'll discuss it more below.

- Illness. Certain diseases such as cancer, as well as the treatments for those diseases, can affect the health of your gums, usually by causing dry mouth. Cancer treatment in particular can cause sores in the mouth that make it painful to brush.
- Genetics. Some people—perhaps 30 percent of the population—are just more genetically susceptible than others to periodontal disease. These people must be absolutely meticulous with their oral hygiene and diet, and usually need regular checkups with their dentist or periodontist.
- Malocclusion. Crooked or crowded teeth, or a bad bite—teeth that don't meet correctly when you bite down—can worsen periodontal disease. (I'll talk more about this later in the chapter.)

Left untreated, periodontal disease leads to pain and lost teeth, but that's only the most obvious result. The invisible damage from periodontal disease affects your whole body.

The Inflammation Connection

Let's say you cut your finger and it gets infected. What happens? It turns red, becomes swollen, feels hot to the touch, and hurts. That's inflammation: redness, swelling, heat, and pain. In the case of your cut finger, inflammation is basically a good thing. Even though it's uncomfortable, it means your body is fighting off the infection.

What if the inflammation was happening inside one of the arteries that nourishes your heart? That wouldn't be such a good thing. Inside an artery, the inflammatory response leads to all sorts of changes—none of them good. The end result of inflammation in your arteries is plaque. That's not the same plaque that can cover your teeth. This type of plaque is a fatty deposit on the inside of the artery. Plaques can become large enough to block off the artery. Or, a piece of plaque can break off, get carried into a smaller blood vessel, and block it. Either way, you end up with a blocked artery. If it cuts off blood flow to your heart, the result is a heart attack; to your brain, a stroke.

So, inflammation is pretty clearly linked to heart disease. And what's a common source of ongoing inflammation in your body? You guessed it—periodontal disease. The same bacteria that cause an immune response leading to red, swollen gums also can get into your circulatory system and cause inflammation in your arteries.

For decades, medical and dental students were taught that patients with bad teeth were more likely to have heart disease. But the direct link was observational, which made it hard to prove. Doctors knew the connection was there, but they couldn't say whether or not the periodontal disease was directly related to the heart disease. Strong as the connection is from observational studies, researchers are still working on proving the link beyond a doubt. People with severe gum disease also tend to be smokers, for instance, so perhaps smoking, not bacteria, is really the link to heart disease.

In recent years, however, several solid studies have gone a long way toward proving the periodontal-heart disease link. One study in 2005[16] showed that people who had higher levels of bacteria in their mouths also had thicker carotid arteries, a well-recognized indicator of heart disease. These people also had a higher risk of stroke. But, the study only showed a connection between high levels of oral bacteria and thicker carotid arteries—it couldn't show which came first.

However, in another 2005 study reported in the prestigious journal *Circulation,*[17] researchers showed that people who had measurable levels of antibodies to the most common bacteria found in periodontitis also had the greatest risk of heart disease—even if they had never smoked. Interestingly, a lot of the participants who had antibodies and heart disease didn't have clinical signs of periodontal disease. In other words, even people in early stages of periodontal disease, before it becomes obvious, were at increased risk of heart disease. This finding is yet another argument for plenty of tooth brushing to prevent gum disease.

An observational study in France in 2007 looked at people who already had both periodontal disease and heart disease.[18] The findings: the worse the periodontal disease, the more serious the heart disease may be. In the study, the patients had x-ray exams of their hearts and coronary blood vessels. All the patients were checked for gum disease and had blood samples taken to check for inflammation markers. Not surprisingly, the patients with the most severe arterial plaque turned out to have the worst periodontitis as well.

What if you already have periodontal disease? Is too late to help your heart? Not at all. In 2007, a study in the *New England Journal of Medicine* showed that intensive treatment of gum disease can lead to improved circulation.[19] In this study, a group of 120 men with severe periodontitis were divided into two groups. Each patient gave a blood sample that was tested for chemical markers of inflammation. Each patient also was tested to see how much the endothelium, or inner lining, of an artery in his arm could open up. The wider the artery could open, the healthier the endothelium, and the better the blood flow. Good endothelial function generally means good heart health, so this was a useful baseline measurement.

The first group of patients received standard care for their gum disease. A dentist scraped and polished their teeth. The second group received more aggressive care. Each patient was given anesthesia to numb his mouth, and a dentist then cleaned away plaque below the gum line and extracted diseased teeth, if necessary.

All the patients were then followed to see what happened to their blood markers and endothelial function. The day after treatment, the patients in the intensive treatment group had higher markers of inflammation and worse endothelial function that those who got standard care. Eight weeks later, however, the intensive treatment group had better results; they were still better six months later. In the long run, then, improved oral health led to improved circulatory health as well.

Another 2007 study published in the *European Journal of Internal*

Medicine followed patients with periodontal disease.[20] *All* patients who received treatment saw their periodontal disease diminish, and laboratory tests confirmed that their arteries became healthier as well! In their conclusions, the authors wrote, "Treating periodontitis can improve endothelial function and be an important preventive tool for cardiovascular disease."

A 2008 article published in the *Journal of Internal Medicine* underlines how important it is to brush your teeth and control periodontal disease. In their conclusion of their 131 patient study, the authors conclude, "…patients might benefit from an intensive periodontal therapy to prevent coronary artery disease progression."[21]

Just as inflammation can lead to a heart attack, so it also can cause a stroke. When plaque breaks off in an artery that leads to your brain, it can block the circulation. Instead of a heart attack, you have a "brain attack"—otherwise known as an ischemic stroke. Treating your periodontal disease can help reduce your risk of both heart attack and stroke.

Periodontal Disease and Diabetes

Almost everyone who has diabetes, especially if it's Type II diabetes (the kind that's related to being overweight and inactive), has a much greater risk of also having periodontal disease. Diabetic patients are often warned that they have an increased risk of heart disease, kidney disease, blindness, and other problems related to high blood sugar. But their increased risk of periodontal disease tends to be ignored. It's real, though, and should get just as much attention as the other potential health problems.

Why does diabetes make you so vulnerable to gum disease? Part of the reason is that diabetes can raise your blood sugar, especially if you don't have the condition under control. We know that diabetics who keep their blood sugar down still get periodontal disease at about the same rate as people without diabetes. So you can see how important good blood sugar control is. The problem is that many people with Type

II diabetes, even the ones who have it under control, have high blood sugar for a long time—often years—before it's finally diagnosed. All that extra sugar in your blood does a lot of damage. In fact, sometimes it's your dentist who will suggest that you might have diabetes.

I am an orthodontist, and all of my new patients must fill out a standard medical history published by the American Dental Association. The history contains questions such as, "How often do you urinate?" and "Are you frequently thirsty?" Often a patient will ask me why I care about these things. What business is it of mine? I'm not being nosy. The answers are important for effective treatment.

Several years ago I began orthodontic treatment on a 47-year-old school teacher. She answered yes to the above questions; she also was overweight and had periodontal disease. I asked her when her last physical was, and if she had ever been tested for diabetes. She hadn't had a checkup in a while, so I sent her to her doctor. Sure enough, she was quickly diagnosed. Her trip to the orthodontist ended up saving her life.

Periodontal disease is an obvious sign of untreated diabetes, but there are other telltale signs as well. Dry mouth, for instance, is often a clue. This can cause mouth sores, tooth decay, and infections. Sore gums from dentures and other dental appliances are another common sign of diabetes.

High blood sugar makes your blood vessels get thicker and less flexible. The smaller the blood vessel, the more damaging that sort of thickening is, because it can clog up the blood flow. That's why diabetes is so damaging to your kidneys and eyes—they're full of tiny blood vessels that are easily damaged. The same is true of your gums. When blood flow in your gums is disrupted, the tissue becomes more vulnerable to infection.

If your blood sugar is high, that means your saliva is high in sugar, too. That's just the sort of mouth environment that infection-causing bacteria love. They'll settle in and start raising very large families inside your gums. You'll need treatment to get rid of the periodontitis they cause, but the treatment won't be as effective as it should be if your blood sugar stays high. Getting your blood sugar under control will help the treatment work and help keep the problem from coming back.

That brings me to an interesting point: high blood sugar can cause periodontal disease, and periodontal disease can raise your blood sugar and make it harder to lower it to a healthier level. We know from experience and a number of studies that treating the periodontal disease can make it easier to keep your blood sugar under control.

In a study published in 2005 in the *Journal of Clinical Periodontology*, two groups of diabetic patients were compared over three months.[22] The study group received complete periodontal care; the control group received none. After three months, the patients who received periodontal care showed a marked improvement in their gums and periodontal health, and their blood sugar levels were improved as well. There was no corresponding improvement in the control group.

In a later study conducted in Spain, similar results were found. The authors concluded, "The diabetic patients showed improved metabolic control at 3 and 6 months after periodontal treatment."[23]

Clear your periodontal disease, and you can help control your diabetes. Once again, treating your mouth treats your whole body.

Healthy Mouth, Healthy Baby

Starting in the 1990s, researchers noticed that pregnant women who had periodontal disease were much more likely to give birth prematurely or to have a baby with low birthweight. Since both problems are serious, and because pregnant women are more susceptible to periodontal disease, this observation got a lot of attention. The next step was to do studies to see if treating periodontal disease during pregnancy would reduce the risk.

Several studies have shown that it does. A 2002 study in Chile showed that the rate of premature birth was only 1.8 percent among a group of women who received periodontal treatment during pregnancy.[24] Among a control group who didn't get treated until after they gave birth, the rate of premature birth was 10.1 percent. A similar study at the same time of women in Alabama had a similar result: the rate of preterm birth in the treated group was 4.1 percent, versus 13.7 percent in the delayed-treatment group.

A follow up to this study, conducted in 2005 yielded the same results. In this study of 870 women, periodontal treatment significantly reduced the number of preterm and low birth weight infants.[25]

Confusing the issue, however, were two major studies that appeared in 2006 and 2007. In the 2006 *New England Journal of Medicine* study, pregnant women who had periodontitis were randomly assigned to have aggressive periodontal treatment during their pregnancy; the other group wasn't treated until after delivery. There wasn't any significant difference between the two groups in the number of premature or low birthweight babies.[26] But a second study, published in the *Journal of Periodontology* in 2007, also compared two groups of pregnant women. In this study, the pregnant women with untreated periodontal disease did have a much higher incidence of preterm babies with low birthweight.[27]

In 2007 the single, largest study ever conducted on this subject was printed. 3,576 women were examined shortly after they gave birth. The researchers noted the mother's periodontal condition, and correlated it to low birthweight outcomes. The results were illuminating. The author's conclusion was simple and direct: "Maternal periodontal disease may be a risk factor for an adverse pregnancy outcome."[28]

The researchers are welcome to argue the question and do more studies, but to me it's perfectly clear: periodontal disease during pregnancy is a bad thing, and treating it promptly is a good thing.

Clean Away Cancer

If reducing your risk of heart attacks, diabetes, and even low birthweight infants isn't enough, here is yet another good reason to brush your teeth: A clean mouth helps to avoid cancer.

Cancers of the mouth, lips, tongue and cheeks are deadly and disfiguring. Proper oral hygiene will help to insure that this horrible disease won't strike you.

Nearly twenty years ago researchers in China discovered that poor oral hygiene was linked to oral cancers. In a study of over 800 people, those individuals who did not brush their teeth were up to 7 times more likely to develop mouth cancers![29] Another study, conducted in Canada with over 2,000 people, yielded similar results. The authors concluded that infrequent tooth brushing is one risk factor for cancer of the mouth.[30]

While it may seem scary that something as simple as not brushing your teeth correctly can cause cancer, the mechanism is simple to understand. Inadequate oral hygiene causes an overgrowth of some pretty obnoxious bacteria. These bacteria (*C. Gingivalis, P. Melaninogenica and Strep mitis*) excrete toxins that cause cavities, periodontal disease and bad breath. The toxins are also carcinogenic, and over a period of time may cause cancer.[31]

The really, really scary part is that these cancer-causing toxins can get into your blood stream and cause cancers in distant organs. In a 16-year study of 51,000 men, those men who had periodontal disease were twice as likely to develop pancreatic cancer. The researchers from Harvard School of Public Health reported that the increased risk of developing pancreatic cancer may occur through "plausible biologic mechanisms," such as bacterial toxins.[32]

Treating Periodontal Disease

You've got periodontitis and it needs to be treated. What happens next?

First, your dentist will assess the problem to see just how bad it really is. The dentist will poke a tiny ruler called a probe down into the pockets around your teeth to see how deep they are. In a healthy mouth, the probe will go in only one to three millimeters; any more than that is almost always a sign of trouble. The dentist also will take x-rays to see if there's any bone loss. Most dentists are comfortable treating mild cases of periodontitis, but for more severe cases you may be referred to a periodontist, a specialist who treats gum disease.

The primary goal of periodontal treatment is to control the infection. There are several ways to do this, but all of them depend to a large degree on the patient. You have to practice good daily dental hygiene at home. If you smoke, your treatment will be a lot more successful if you quit.

Treating periodontal disease begins with deep cleaning—scaling and root planning—to remove plaque and tartar. Scaling means scraping off the tartar that has formed above and below the gum line. Root planing smoothes out rough spots on the tooth root where bacteria accumulate. To help your body fight off the infection, your dentist also may recommend antibiotic medication. The medication, usually in the form of a "chip" or gel, is placed directly into the pocket, where it is slowly released over several days. The antibiotic controls bacteria and reduces the size of the pocket.

Even after scaling, root planing, and antibiotics, inflammation and deep pockets may still remain. In that case, your dentist or periodontist may recommend surgical treatment. If you thought deep cleaning was fun, you'll love gum surgery. It generally involves lifting back the gums, removing the tartar, and then suturing the gum back into place so that the tissue fits tightly around the teeth again. In really severe cases, you might need a bone or tissue graft to help regrow bone or gum tissue that has been destroyed by periodontitis.

Brush Your Teeth! And Floss!

I hope that after reading all the problems that periodontal disease can cause, you're ready to start paying a bit more attention to your dental hygiene. A few extra minutes with your toothbrush every day could save you many long hours in the dentist's chair. And in addition to having a nicer smile, you'll be helping your overall health.

I'm an orthodontist, which means a lot of my patients are wearing braces and other dental appliances. That means they have to brush their teeth—*a lot.* Years of experience have taught me that most of my pa-tients need a refresher course in the best way to keep their teeth clean.

I am amazed by how many children simply don't brush their teeth. They come into my office with food and plaque and globs of bacte-ria stuck in between their teeth. I ask, "When was the last time you brushed your teeth?" "This morning," they answer. I say to them, "You may have put a toothbrush somewhere near your mouth and moved it around a bit, but believe me, you haven't brushed your teeth."

Then I do this demonstration: I give patients a mirror and show them the globs of gooey, whitish plaque hugging their teeth. I get a toothbrush into position and ask an assistant to give me a time check. She counts, "One one-thousand, two one-thousand, three one-thou-sand …" By the time she gets to "five one-thousand" I have thoroughly cleaned the front surface of the six front teeth! Sure, cleaning the whole mouth takes a little longer, but this demonstration clearly shows that no real attempt has been made at brushing for quite a while.

The first step in good tooth-brushing is to select a good toothbrush. There are dozens of brands from which to choose, with all sorts of shapes to the heads and handles and all sorts of claims of being the best at cleaning your teeth. Which brand you choose doesn't really matter. Select a brush that fits your hand comfortably so that you'll be comfort-able while brushing. The best toothbrush in the world won't help you much if you don't use it! Look for soft bristles—just about all tooth-brushes today have them. Once you find a style you like, buy several. Your toothbrush should be replaced at least every three months. Many of my patients like electric toothbrushes. Most of these have timers, which help you brush for as long as you should. The heads for electric toothbrushes are more expensive than regular toothbrushes, but don't cheap out—replace them at least every three months.

Toothbrushes, in a sense, have been around in various forms since before recorded history. Chewsticks of various nature, tree twigs, bird feathers, animal bones and porcupine quills have all been used as a tool for oral hygiene. The first modern style toothbrush was a Chinese invention in the late 15th century. Stiff hairs from a hog's neck were attached to a bamboo stick.

The first patent for a toothbrush was by H. N. Wadsworth in 1857 (US Patent No. 18,653) in the United States. The patent shows a bone handle with holes bored into it for the Siberian Boar hair bristles. But Boar isn't an ideal material; it retains bacteria, doesn't dry well, and the bristles tend to fall out of the brush.

DuPont replaced animal hair bristles with nylon in 1938. The Bristol-Myers Company (now Bristol-Myers Squibb) introduced the first electric toothbrush, the Broxodent, at the meeting of the American Dental Association in 1959.

In 2003 the toothbrush was selected as the number one invention Americans could not live without, beating out the automobile, computer, cell phone, and microwave oven, according to the Lemelson-MIT Invention Index.

As with toothbrushes, so with toothpastes. Today there's a bewildering variety of them out there. Choose one with fluoride. The rest is up to your personal taste. If you're fighting periodontal disease, your dentist may recommend toothpaste with the antibiotic triclosan. If you have sensitive teeth, there are many desensitizing toothpastes that can help. You may want to choose a toothpaste with a whitening agent.

OK, it's time to brush your teeth. Why are you doing this again? To remove food particles, stimulate your gums, and keep plaque from building up.

Put some toothpaste on your toothbrush. Ready? The key is to have a plan and a pattern. It's not haphazard. Start with the molars all the way at the back of your mouth—top or bottom, left side or right, it doesn't really matter. Hold your brush against the outer surface (the cheek side) of the back molar at the gum line at a 45-degree angle. Jiggle the brush in a small circular motion five or six times. Remember that you are not scrubbing the kitchen floor here! The bristles shouldn't jump from tooth to tooth. Instead, you're aiming to jiggle them into the crevices between the teeth. Use light pressure— you shouldn't feel discomfort. Clean two or three teeth at a time. Next, move the brush forward a bit in your mouth and repeat. Follow this until you get to the other side of your jaw. Repeat this procedure on the opposite jaw, then on the inside surfaces of the teeth.

To clean the chewing surfaces of your molars, hold the brush head horizontally and move it back and forth while pressing down a bit to get the bristles down into the grooves of the teeth. To clean the backs of your top and bottom front teeth, turn the brush so you can use the tip to get into this narrower area. The whole process should take you a couple of minutes. If it takes less, chances are you're skimping by not brushing each area long enough. Brush longer, not harder.

When you're done with your teeth, gently brush your tongue. This helps get rid of the bacteria that accumulate on the tongue's surface. Reach back with your toothbrush as far as you can without gagging, and gently brush forward about half a dozen times.

Now comes the next step: flossing. You could brush your teeth for 20 minutes and you still wouldn't remove the bits of food and plaque that are between your teeth and under the gum line. That's where dental floss—a strong, thin filament designed to fit between your teeth—comes in. Flossing gets in between the teeth and down below the gum line to scrape out the debris.

Using dental floss properly is important, because incorrect use can damage your gums. The crucial thing here is to be gentle but thorough.

Start with a piece of dental floss about 18 inches long. Wrap one end securely around the index or middle finger of one hand. Then wrap the other end around the index or middle finger of the other hand. You should have about five inches of floss in between. Pinch that length of floss between the thumb and index finger of each hand so that there's only about an inch between them. Starting with the back molars on one side (top or bottom, left or right, whichever you prefer), gently slide the floss in between two teeth, using a seesaw motion to get it all the way down to the gum. Don't force the floss down or yank on it—you could damage your gums. Curve the floss into a C shape around the first tooth, then move it gently up and down to scrape the tooth and clean it. Curve the floss in the opposite direction and repeat on the other tooth. Remove the floss. If the floss gets stuck on the way out, don't yank up on it—let go of one end of the floss and pull it out through the teeth instead. Repeat the process with the next pair of teeth. Unwrap more clean floss from your fingers as you need it.

Some people can't (or won't) use dental floss. Fortunately, there are alternative methods for cleaning in between teeth that are just as effective as floss. These devices are called interproximal toothbrushes or interdental cleaners. They're like toothpicks with an attitude! They are designed to clean the same areas as dental floss. Many people find them far easier to use, and are thus more likely to incorporate them into their everyday oral hygiene.

Beyond Brushing

Antimicrobial mouth rinses. These have recently gained official acceptance by the American Dental Association.[33] In at least 30 clinical studies, such mouth rinses have been proven to help prevent and reduce plaque and gingivitis. In fact, adding an antiseptic mouth rinse to a routine of brushing and flossing can kill up to 50 percent more bacteria than can brushing and flossing alone. If used properly, a rinse can reach the whole mouth, killing germs in "reservoirs" where plaque bacteria survive. This is especially true for patients who are older or physically impaired and may not have the dexterity to brush and floss effectively.

Make sure you rinse properly. Brush and floss first, then swish the liquid around vigorously through your teeth for 30 seconds. Clock yourself the first few times. These mouth rinses tend to sting, and 15 seconds may seem like a minute!

Diet. If you brush and floss your teeth twice a day, can you eat all the candy you want? Nope. Sugary foods are the number-one cause of tooth decay and periodontal disease. If you include a lot of these foods (and drinks) in your diet, all the dental hygiene in the world won't be enough to prevent problems. The top sugar culprit is carbonated soft drinks. One serving can include 11 or more teaspoons of sugar![34] Your intake of candies, cakes, and all other foods that are high in sugars and simple carbohydrates should also be limited. I'll talk a lot more about diet in a later chapter. For now, let's just say that for the sake of your teeth—as well as your waistline and overall health—stay away from high-sugar, low-nutrient foods.

Certain nutrients can make a big difference in your oral health. These include calcium, magnesium, vitamin C, and vitamin D. You need all four, especially calcium, to build bones that will stay strong as you get older. Osteoporosis can result in bone loss in the jaw. This, in turn, can make your teeth shift or even loosen, which can lead to periodontal disease and other big dental problems. A study published in the *Journal of Periodontology* showed that calcium deficiency could lead to a 54 percent increase in periodontal disease.[35]

Going hand-in-hand with calcium is vitamin D, another nutrient required for bone health. Your body actually can manufacture vitamin D through exposure to sunlight. But increases in indoor activities and necessary use of sunscreen lotions, coupled with decreased consumption of milk, mean more and more people are deficient in vitamin D.

Vitamin C, or ascorbic acid, also is crucial for gum and bone health. In one major study, researchers analyzed vitamin C intakes and periodontal-disease indicators in 12,000 adults.[36] Patients who consumed less than the recommended 60 milligrams (mg) per day of vitamin C—about the amount in one orange—had nearly one-and-a-half times the risk of developing severe gingivitis compared to those who consumed the most vitamin C.

Vitamin C helps maintain the integrity of the small capillaries. These supply blood and nutrients to your tissues and organs, including your gums. Inadequate consumption of vitamin C causes the capillaries of the gums and mouth to degenerate. This was discovered more than 250 years ago when doctors realized that scurvy, a disease caused by lack of vitamin C, could be cured with citrus fruit. Yet even today, as much as 20 percent of the American public is still deficient in vitamin C.

Prevention is the best strategy here. I strongly recommend that all my patients, from teenagers on up, take a daily calcium supplement with added vitamin D and magnesium.

Melatonin. Although melatonin is a hormone mostly associated with sleep, it may be an important factor in periodontal disease as well. It enters the blood during sleep, and studies have proven that people who get inadequate sleep are more likely to suffer periodontal disease. Melatonin also is released into the saliva and may have important implications for periodontal health.[37] Melatonin has powerful antioxidant effects and promotes bone formation. It also stimulates the immune system as well as the synthesis of collagen fibers, which are the building blocks of gum tissue,.

Crooked teeth. Most people—even many dentists—are not fully aware that crooked teeth can cause periodontal disease. Crooked or crowded teeth are far more difficult to keep clean and will collect far more plaque and tartar. Toothbrush bristles can't negotiate the deep crevices caused by crowded, overlapping teeth. Furthermore, the crowding causes different, more virulent, more destructive bacteria to live in the gums. Fortunately, braces or *Invisalign®* clear aligners can almost always correct crowding!

*Invisalign®*is a method of orthodontic therapy for straightening teeth without using traditional braces. Instead of metal braces, a series of clear, custom-fabricated aligners are designed to gradually and sequentially move teeth to their desired positions. The most obvious advantage of the treatment is cosmetic: the aligners are completely transparent and more difficult to detect. This makes the method particularly popular among adults who want to straighten their teeth without the look of traditional metal braces commonly worn by children. In addition, the aligners are more comfortable than braces. Since *Invisalign®*aligners are removable, there are no eating restrictions.

*Invisalign®*is particularly advantageous for patients with periodontal disease. Because they are removable, they don't act as "food traps," and it is far easier to maintain adequate oral hygiene. Average treatment time is about one year, depending on the complexity of the problem. Treatment of minor crowding or minor spacing may take less time.

Orthodontic treatment can not only make your smile look better, it will help to control periodontal disease.

Take Your Gums Seriously

I don't think people take periodontal disease seriously enough. It is not a benign problem limited to just bleeding gums. Perhaps if we renamed the disease, and called it what it really is, people would treat it with more determination. It's not just periodontal disease: it's a *Putrid, Festering Infection of the Mouth!*

Now that's serious!

CHAPTER 2

Wash Your Hands

If there's just one simple idea for improving your health—and the health of those around you—it's this: wash your hands.

I'm sure this isn't a new idea to you. In fact, it's something you've probably been hearing for as long as you can remember. You don't have to think back very hard to your childhood to hear your mother saying to you, "Just look at those hands! Go wash them." You probably don't have to think much harder to remember just about every other adult in your life saying the same thing at some point.

Why did the grown-ups keep making you wash your hands? Why should you probably wash your hands even more than you already do? Why should you encourage all those around you to wash their hands frequently as well? Because infectious diseases, many of which are easily spread by dirty hands, cause millions of Americans to miss school or work each week.[38] Furthermore, infectious diseases remain the third leading cause of death in the United States, right behind heart attacks and cancer.

The numbers are really eye-opening:

- Every year, according to the CDC, there are more than 52 million cases of the common cold just among Americans younger than age 17. In fact, the average child today catches a cold about six to ten times a year. If you have a few children, all in school or daycare, the average number of colds they'll catch goes up to twelve a year.

- Colds alone account for 22 million lost school days.
- Adults, with their stronger immune systems, still catch an average of two to four colds a year.
- During flu season—usually November to March—about 10 to 20 percent of all Americans catch the flu. Most people recover after a couple of weeks of coughing and feeling lousy, but every year about 100,000 people need to be hospitalized, and about 36,000 die from flu or its complications.
- Children are two to three times more likely than adults to come down with the flu.
- Poor hand washing, or not washing at all, accounts for nearly half of foodborne illness outbreaks. Millions of people get sick each year from foodborne illness, and about 5,000 people a year in the United States die from foodborne illness caused by bacteria such as salmonella or campylobacter.[39]

Makes you want to put this book down and go wash your hands, doesn't it?

Germs, Microbes and Superbugs

About 80 percent of all infectious diseases, including colds, flu, and gastrointestinal infections, are transmitted by touch.[40] You touch something that's contaminated with dangerous microbes; then you touch your face—usually your mouth, nose, or eyes. The germs enter your body, where they can cause illness. And if you're sick—even if you don't feel sick—you pass those germs on every time you touch something.

But before we go any further, you should know exactly what I mean by the terms "germs" and "microbes." These are general terms for all kinds of microorganisms, or very tiny life forms. These include bacteria, such as the ones that cause salmonella; viruses, such as the ones that cause colds and flu; fungi, such as the ones that cause athlete's foot; and even parasites, such as the ones that cause giardia, an intestinal ailment.

Most bacteria aren't harmful, and in fact, some are even helpful. You rely on some kinds of bacteria in your intestines, for instance, to manufacture vitamin K, which is essential for blood clotting and strong bones.

Harmful germs, however, are another story. They multiply really, really fast. When conditions are right—which usually means warm and wet—a single bacteria cell can grow and divide every 20 minutes. If you do the math, you'll realize that this means one invisibly small germ cell can become more than 8 million cells in just 24 hours. So, one harmful germ cell that lands on your hand and stays there even for a few hours may multiply into many thousands. When you then prepare food without first washing your hands, those bacteria get into the food—and also onto the kitchen counter, the kitchen towel, the knife handle, and anything else you touch. They might even get into you if you cut or scratch yourself. What it comes down is this: your unwashed hands are an infection waiting to happen.

Microorganisms, including harmful ones, are always around us—they're a normal part of our environment. And if you're a healthy adult, most of the time your immune system will destroy any harmful germs that enter your body before they have a chance to make you sick. But even the healthiest person doesn't have a perfectly efficient immune system—and some germs can be so virulent that your immune system can't react in time to keep you from getting sick. Children have immature immune systems that can't respond well to infectious diseases, which is why they get sick so easily with illnesses that generally don't bother adults. Similarly, older adults have immune systems that don't react as quickly as they used to, which makes them more vulnerable to illness. And anyone with an impaired immune system is also a lot more vulnerable to infectious disease. Someone who's getting chemotherapy to treat cancer, for instance, needs to be very careful about avoiding infection. The same applies to anyone with an ongoing illness such as HIV/AIDS, chronic bronchitis, or multiple sclerosis, to name just a few. And even healthy adults go through times of being so busy or so stressed—or both—that they don't get enough sleep, don't eat right, and make themselves more vulnerable to infectious disease.

An even greater concern is the growing problem of drug-resistant "superbugs"—bacteria that can't be killed even by the most powerful antibiotics. These bacteria are known as methicillin-resistant *Staphylococcus aureus*, or MRSA. Most people who become infected with MRSA are hospital patients. The latest research suggests that nearly 5 percent of all hospital patients who carry the bacteria, die from it.[41] Recently, however, there have been more cases of MRSA spreading through public schools and athletic teams. And what's the number-one way to keep these deadly bacteria from spreading to other patients in the hospital? Hand washing. That means *everybody* in the hospital, not just the staff. Patients and the people who visit them need to wash often and well. Today many hospitals and nursing homes place dispensers containing hand-sanitizing gel near all the entrances. Visitors are encouraged to use them. If you don't see a dispenser, find a washroom and wash with soap and water before you visit someone.

A 2007 study published in the *British Medical Journal Website* says it all: "Physical barriers" such as handwashing are more effective than drugs or vaccines in preventing the spread of respiratory viruses such as influenza.[42]

How Germs Spread

For germs to spread from one person to another, there has to be some sort of contact, either direct or indirect. Direct transmission occurs when you touch another person: you shake hands, hug, or kiss, for example. Indirect transmission occurs when you touch something that has previously been touched, such as a computer keyboard, telephone, or doorknob. In either case, touching brings you into contact with germs.

Think of it this way: every time you touch a handrail, pen, elevator button, or vending machine, you're infecting yourself with the mucous, spit, sweat, and germs of the last hundred people who did the same! Or, if you're the sick one, you're leaving behind germs that others may catch.

Breaking that chain of transmission is clearly the most effective way to prevent illness. And what's the best way to break the chain? Wash your hands—often.

It's an obvious message, and one that's probably been drilled into you since childhood, yet it turns out that an awful lot of us haven't been paying attention. In 2006, the people who make *Lysol* did a worldwide survey of handwashing habits. Even allowing for the fact that the manufacturers wanted to sell more *Lysol* products, the results were pretty shocking. Two-thirds of the people surveyed knew that handwashing is the best way to stop the spread of germs, but at the same time, sixty-seven percent of those surveyed admitted that they didn't always wash their hands when they should, such as after sneezing or coughing, or after handling animals or pets.

Other surveys have found that people just don't wash their hands as often as they think (or say) that they do. In one survey, 94 percent of all adults said they washed their hands after using the bathroom.[43] But based on data from hidden cameras viewing more than six thousand adults using public restrooms in five big American cities, only about 68 percent actually washed their hands. In other words, only about two out of three washed, which means that about a third of all the people observed in the study didn't. And even though children hear the handwashing message all day long, it still doesn't always get through. In a study reported in the *American Journal of Infection Control,* only 58 percent of girls and 48 percent of boys in middle school and high school washed their hands after using the bathroom.[44]

And that's—yuck—after using the bathroom. How many people do you think routinely wash their hands before they eat? Almost nobody!

Why People Don't Wash Their Hands

Most people don't routinely wash their hands for three simple reasons.

1. Lack of noticeable cause and effect.

Imagine training your dog to sit down and give you his paw. You would give the dog the command, "sit, paw," gently push his butt down, take his paw, and then reward him with a treat. You would do this several times, each time rewarding the dog for good behavior.

But what if you didn't reward the dog immediately after the good behavior? What if you gave him the treat two or three days later? Do you think the dog would connect the good behavior to the treat? Of course not.

When people don't wash routinely—before eating, touching their faces, scratching their eyes or noses—they may be infecting themselves with germs. If they immediately came down with a cold, flu, or stomach infection each time they skipped washing, they would soon learn to avoid this bad behavior. However, illness caused by not washing appropriately doesn't show up until several days later—sometimes not at all. Most people never connect the dots. They don't realize the cold they are suffering through now was caused by poor hand hygiene several days ago.

2. Most of the time, nothing happens.

Most of us don't routinely follow proper hand hygiene, yet most of the time nothing happens. We eat meals 21 times a week and snack dozens more times during the same period. We touch our faces hundreds of times a week. Usually nothing happens, so we learn that it's OK to cheat now and then and not wash properly.

This sense of false security is dangerous. Most of the time when you drive somewhere, you don't get into an accident; yet it would be foolish (and illegal) to drive without putting on your seat belt. Most of the time when you go to sleep at night, you wake up the next morning safe and sound; yet it would be dangerous not to have a working smoke detector "just in case."

It's exactly the same with proper hygiene. You never know when your fingers have picked up a bad bug. The only way to be safe is to wash your hands frequently.

3. Engineering barriers.

I was recently at a large health-care convention in Las Vegas with more than 1,000 other health-care workers. There were physicians and dentists, nurses and hygienists. After the wrap-up session, there was a large cocktail reception in the huge ballroom next door. After sitting for an hour and a half in the lecture hall, we were all ready to party! All of us human beings were sitting there after coughing and scratching, blowing our noses, and shaking each other's hands.

When the lecture finally ended, the doors opened and we piled out. The throngs of people walked down the hall and into the next ballroom, where we dined on miniature pizza-bagels, mozzarella sticks, "lamb pops," cheese and crackers, nuts, and other delightful finger foods and crudités.

We were all health-care workers—people who wash our hands for a living. We're expert hand-washers. Yet few of us at that conference made the detour to go down the hall in the opposite direction to wash our hands. It was too inconvenient, and the bathrooms would not have supported so many people at a time. Public health officials call this an "engineering barrier." They're everywhere.

When my oldest daughter was visiting colleges a couple of years ago, we took a family trip to visit an Ivy League school. As is our practice during all of our college visits, we ate lunch at one of the college cafeterias. At the entrance, we paid the meal fee, and asked where the restrooms were.

"Go down the hall to the end and turn left. It's halfway down on the right," the cashier informed us.

We journeyed down to visit the restroom, and were surprised to find that it was a single washroom. No men's room, no women's room—just a unisex room with a toilet and sink. Clearly, the architects and engineers who designed this dining hall didn't plan for proper hand-washing.

These Ivy League students spend the mornings exchanging germs by touching desks and chairs and doorknobs and books and *Frisbees*, and then high-fiving each other before having their midday meal. They don't have an easy way to wash their hands before they eat—so they don't. Could it be any clearer why colds and flu and stomach viruses spread like wildfire through college campuses?

How to Wash Your Hands

You wouldn't think that adults would need to be taught how to wash their hands, but you'd be surprised. In fact, the first lesson in any school for health professionals is: how to wash your hands.

I attended graduate school at Columbia University Health Science Center. My first course was gross anatomy, where medical and dental students learned anatomy by dissecting cadavers. There were four students assigned to each cadaver. (We named our cadaver "Abra." That would be Abra Cadaver.) We cut and sliced and dissected the body until we could fit every piece of the body through a baseball-sized hole. The stink of formaldehyde permeated the air and was absorbed by our skin and clothing.

The course went from 9:00 AM until noon. Lunch was immediately after. You can be sure we learned how to wash our hands!

So, pretend you're a medical student on the first day of class. Here's how to wash your hands:

- Wash your hands with soap and clean running water for at least 20 seconds. How long is 20 seconds? Just about long enough to sing the alphabet song to yourself. If you get tired of that song, sing the birthday song twice or sing a verse of "Twinkle,

Twinkle, Little Star." If you're in the holiday spirit, try the chorus of "Jingle Bells."

- Warm water is best, if it's available, because it helps soap emulsify normal skin oils and grease, but cold water will work fine, too. Don't use water that's as hot as you can stand—the water would have to be near boiling to kill any more germs than cold water, and the risk of scalding is too great.
- Rub your hands together to make a lather, then scrub your hands all over—top and bottom, between the fingers, across the knuckles, under the nails, and up over your wrists. Friction is important here. It forces the lather deep into the crevices of your skin and helps in the emulsification process, plus it helps to dislodge germs and sloughed skin cells.
- Rinse your hands thoroughly under running water.
- Dry your hands using a paper towel or a clean cloth towel. An equally good choice is the air dryer if you're in a public restroom that has one.
- If you use a paper towel to dry, also use it to turn off the faucet.

Washing for 20 seconds is a crucial part of the process. Any less, and you won't be removing as many germs as you could. But washing for much more than 20 seconds won't remove many more germs, so unless you're about to do surgery, you don't have to wash any longer than that.

Twenty seconds seems to be too long for a lot of people. A 2006 study by the Soap and Detergent Association found that while more than half of all adults surveyed washed their hands several times a day, at least half did so for less than 20 seconds.[45]

When to Wash Your Hands

The short answer to when to wash your hands is as often as possible. More specifically, be sure to wash your hands at all these times:

- Before eating
- Before preparing food and immediately after handling raw food, such as raw chicken
- Before and after tending to someone who's sick
- Before and after treating a cut or wound
- Before giving or taking medicine
- Before putting in contact lenses
- After going to the bathroom
- After blowing your nose, coughing, or sneezing
- After changing diapers
- After cleaning up a child who has gone to the bathroom
- After handling an animal or animal waste, such as after cleaning the litter box
- After handling any sort of blood or body fluids, such as saliva or vomit
- After handling garbage or anything else that might be contaminated, such as a sink drain
- After being in a public place, such as the supermarket or the movies
- After being outside, such as in the garden or at the playground with the kids
- After touching money. A 2008 study from the National Influenza Research Centre at Geneva University Hospital reports that flu and other viruses can survive on paper money for up to 17 days![46]
- Whenever your hands look dirty

That's a really long list, and I could make it even longer. I don't need to, though, because it all comes back to one simple thing: wash your hands—often.

Selecting Soap

When I was a kid, there wasn't any question about what sort of soap to use. Plain old bar soap was pretty much all there was. Times have changed, though, and today you have a lot of soap options. What's best? Plain old bar soap, it turns out, isn't the first choice. That's because the bar itself can end up harboring germs from the different people who use it. A better choice is an antibacterial soap. The antibacterial agent in bar soaps is usually triclocarban; in some bar soaps and in liquid soaps, it's triclosan. Both are safe and effective antimicrobial ingredients. Triclosan has been in widespread use for more than 30 years.

Generally speaking, antibacterial soaps are more effective than plain soap because the triclosan- or triclocarban-and-soap combo kills more germs than soap alone. More importantly, antibacterial soap reduces the number of germs on your skin for up to several hours after washing. These soaps kill or inhibit the bacteria that cause odor, skin infections, food poisoning, and intestinal illnesses. They're also helpful against the viruses that cause stomach upsets, colds, and flu. Among antibacterial soaps, liquid soap is more sanitary and more convenient than bar soap. All you have to do is give your hands a quick squirt, and you're ready to start your 20- second song.

You may be concerned that use of antibacterial soaps can lead to increased antibiotic resistance on the part of germs. This is one worry you can forget about. It's true that overuse of antibiotic drugs, such as penicillin and tetracycline, does create antibiotic resistance among bacteria. But antibiotic soaps don't act in the same way as antibiotic drugs. The triclosan in antibacterial soap acts across a broad spectrum of bacteria, as opposed to the narrow range targeted by antibiotic drugs. This means the bacteria can't develop resistance to triclosan. The FDA and a number of scientific studies have looked at triclosan pretty closely, and the conclusion is that using antibacterial soap doesn't create superbugs.[47]

What about all those scented, non-antibacterial soaps in pretty colors and shapes? Use them, by all means. Anything that makes you enjoy washing your hands is good. These soaps are fun, so they're also a good way to get children into the habit of hand washing.

Soap and Water Alternatives

Considering the long list of times when you should wash your hands, you might think that you should never be more than about 10 feet away from a fully equipped bathroom. Life isn't always that convenient, however, and there will always be times when you should wash your hands, but are nowhere near a bathroom.

Fortunately, there's an easy solution to that problem. (If only all health problems could be solved so easily!) Hand-sanitizing gels work almost as well as soap and water. They're convenient, quick, effective, and safe. Alcohol is the most common germ-killing ingredient, but these products also may contain benzalkonium chloride or benzethonium chloride. Both are safe and effective germ killers.[48]

For maximum germ-killing, sanitizing gels need to be used correctly:

- Apply one or two squirts of the gel to the palm of one hand.
- Rub your hands together briskly.
- Rub the gel all over your hands, just as if you were washing them. Be sure to get between the fingers and around and under the nails.
- Keep rubbing until your hands are dry—about 20 seconds.

Gels are handy and effective, but they're designed chiefly to kill germs, not to clean. In other words, if your hands are visibly dirty, use the gel only if you really can't get to a sink. It will help, but it won't get your hands as clean as if you washed.

In hospitals, staff members are told to use the gel before and after any patient contact, but to wash with soap and water if they get anything such as blood on their hands. Staff members actually prefer the gels, because they're quick and easy to use. They also like them because they cause less skin irritation than soap and warm water. Given how often health-care workers must wash their hands over the course of a shift, that's an important consideration.

If you do get skin irritation from a sanitizing gel, it could be from the active ingredient, an added perfume, or a coloring agent, not from the gel itself. Try a different brand, or choose a clear, fragrance-free gel. Clear gels also can help you avoid clothing stains that can occur with tinted gels.

Because sanitizing gels are so convenient, they've made a real improvement in hand sanitation in places like hospitals and doctors' offices. They also can be really helpful in schools. I know this because my daughter is responsible for getting gel dispensers installed by the lunchroom entrance in her school. She complained that she had to go all the way down a long hall in the opposite direction of the school cafeteria so that she could wash her hands in the girls' bathroom before lunch. The time this took was making her late, so my daughter borrowed an idea from a recent family cruise-ship vacation. The cruise line, in a valiant attempt to cut down on shipboard illness, installed sanitizing gel dispensers all throughout the ship. In fact, each entrance to the dining room was manned by an employee with a sanitizing gel dispenser.

My daughter thought, why not install sanitizing gel dispensers by the school lunchroom entrance? That way everyone could have clean hands before eating. She brought the idea up with the school superintendent, whose response was, "That's a real no-brainer." The dispensers went up a few weeks later.

I don't know if the gels made a difference in how often the students got sick at my daughter's school. But, a 2000 study of hand gels in elementary schools did. In the study, students and teachers used hand gel every time they entered or left the classroom. Absenteeism among the students dropped by nearly 20 percent—and by about 10 percent among the teachers.[49] When you compare the cost of paying substitute teachers to the cost of buying some hand-gel dispensers, it really is a no-brainer

Sanitizing gel can have a real health impact at home, too. In 2004, a study by Harvard Medical School compared families who used sanitizer gel with families who didn't. Gel-users had a 59 percent reduction in the spread of gastrointestinal illnesses.[50] In other words, when one family member came down with an intestinal bug, more than half the time it didn't get passed on to other family members. The gel also cut down on the number of colds in the family, though that effect wasn't as dramatic.

The Harvard study was called "Healthy Hands, Healthy Families," and appeared in the prestigious medical journal *Pediatrics.* For the study, researchers recruited nearly three hundred families who had at least one child in day care. Half the families carried on as usual, but the other half received plenty of bottles of hand sanitizer and were told to put them around the house in convenient places, such as the kitchen and the baby's room. The difference in family health was pretty clear after just five months.

The study got a fair amount of attention when it came out, and of course the manufacturers of the gels jumped on it and started offering all sorts of gel products. One day two of my young patients arrived with their mother. Both boys were wearing little gel dispensers attached to their belts. Young boys aren't noted for their interest in sanitation, so I was a little surprised. Their mother noticed my reaction and was quick to tell me that the boys had seen the dispensers in the store and asked for them. She didn't want me to think she was some sort of clean freak. I told her I thought the boys would get over the novelty of it all pretty quickly, and they did. At their next appointment a few weeks later, the gel dispensers were gone. But I was happy to hear that they still used the dispensers at home and at school.

I was amazed recently to get an e-mail warning me about the "dangers" of alcohol hand sanitizer. Supposedly, children have been licking their hands after using the gels and getting poisoned from the alcohol. I guess it's possible that something of the sort might have happened to some child somewhere, but this is really just an urban myth. Obviously no child (or adult, for that matter) should be swallowing the gel; but, when used properly, there's no gel left on your hands after you rub it in—the alcohol evaporates. Common sense applies here. Use the gels according to the directions, and keep the containers out of the reach of small children.

When your hands are really dirty but you can't wash conveniently, disposable wipes are a good option. They get the dirt off and kill germs, though not as effectively as washing or using gel. Just wipe your hands all over until they look clean. Use more than one wipe if you need to, and let your hands air dry. Unless you want a plumber's bill, don't flush wipes! Instead, dispose of used wipes in a trash can.

Beyond Hand Washing

OK, you've decided to wash your hands a lot more. Good decision.

Now it's time to take a few more easy steps that will improve the cleanliness of your environment—your home, your workplace, your school. These measures are surprisingly simple and amazingly effective in cutting back on illness. Follow them, and you and your family will be healthier overall, with fewer lost work and school days.

Kitchen Safety

When my grandmother wanted to compliment someone's housekeeping, she would say, "You could eat off her floors." Before I get started on the importance of good kitchen hygiene, let me just say that I don't recommend eating off the floor. Important as household hygiene is, it's also important to keep it all in perspective. You don't have to be a fanatical neat freak in order to have a safe, sanitary kitchen and home. Just apply the ideas in this chapter in a commonsense way, and you'll have a healthier home without spending a lot of extra time and energy.

Let's start with why kitchen hygiene is so important. Generally speaking, the kitchen is the center of family life. Not only is it where food is stored, prepared, and eaten, it's also where family members come together—along with friends, pets, and just about anyone else who comes into the house. It's a hard place to keep clean, as anyone who has seen dirty footprints tracking across a just-washed floor can tell you.

Because the kitchen is such a popular place, it's pretty obvious that it's also the most likely place for illnesses to be passed around as people come together. What many people may not realize, however, is that the kitchen can be the source of illnesses that can be traced back to food storage and preparation.

Foodborne Disease

There are more than 250 different foodborne diseases. Most of them are rare, however, so there's really only a handful you have to worry about:

- *Salmonella.* The *Salmonella* bacterium is normally found in the intestines of healthy birds, reptiles, and mammals. OK, humans are mammals, too, but in us, *Salmonella* causes an illness known as salmonellosis, or more commonly, food poisoning. The chief symptoms are diarrhea, abdominal cramps, and fever.
- *Campylobacter.* This bacterium is the most common cause of diarrheal illness in the world. Because it's normally found in the intestines of healthy birds, just about all raw poultry has *Campylobacter* on it.
- *Escherichia coli* O157:H7. This is an especially dangerous form of the common bacterium *E. coli.* Healthy people have literally billions of *E. coli* in their intestines, but the O157:H7 form is found mostly in cattle. Beef and other red meats contaminated by this form can make humans very sick. Symptoms include severe bloody diarrhea and abdominal cramps.
- Norwalk viruses, also called norovirus. This is a catchall term for several different viruses that cause vomiting and sometimes diarrhea. Norwalk-virus illnesses generally come on suddenly but last only a couple of days, so they're often assumed to be just a "stomach bug" you picked up somewhere. In fact, Norwalk

virus is passed on when someone who has the virus—but probably doesn't realize it—prepares food that someone else eats. You also can spread the virus if you touch surfaces or objects contaminated with it, then place your hands in your mouth. You've probably heard of this one, because norovirus is the bug responsible for outbreaks of gastrointestinal illness on college campuses and cruise ships.

Foodborne illnesses cause a lot of damage—and not just ruined vacations. According to the CDC (the people who keep track of these things), about 76 million (yes, *million*) cases of foodborne illness occur each year in the United States. That works out to one in four Americans every year. Most cases are mild, of course, but every year about 325,000 people need hospitalization for a foodborne illness; of those, about 5,000 will die.[51] Babies and young children, the elderly, and people with compromised immune systems are most vulnerable.

Preventing foodborne disease is clearly pretty important. And what's the first step for stopping these illnesses? You guessed it: wash your hands. Always wash both before and after handling food. Because raw meats, poultry, seafood, and eggs are the most likely sources of bacteria, it's especially important to wash your hands after handling these items.

The next steps are just as easy and commonsense:

- Check foods before you buy them. In particular, make sure that refrigerated foods have been kept refrigerated. Don't buy precut items, such as melons or prepackaged salads, if you have doubts about how cold they've been kept.
- Clean everything. That's so important I'll get into it in more detail later in this chapter.
- Separate foods. Keep fresh fruits and vegetables separate from raw meat, poultry, and seafood. Keep them apart in your shopping cart, in bags at the checkout, and in the fridge when you

get home. Store meat, poultry, and seafood at the bottom of the fridge, preferably in the meat drawer, so that juices from the packaging can't drip onto other foods. Most important of all: keep fresh meat, poultry, and seafood separate during food preparation. If you're using a cutting board to slice up chicken, for instance, wash it in hot, soapy water before chopping vegetables on it. (Or better yet, have more than one cutting board so you're not tempted to cheat.) If vegetables or fruits have touched raw meat, poultry, or seafood, either cook them right away or throw them out.

- Chill foods. I don't mean tell them to relax. I mean get fresh foods into the fridge or freezer as soon as possible. Bacteria don't grow well in the dry, cold refrigerator or freezer, but they just love warm, moist places, such as a package of meat left out on the counter for a few hours. When you're shopping for groceries, purchase your perishables last. Pack all of the cold items together so they'll stay cold longer. I like to use an inexpensive, insulated storage bag that I bought at the supermarket for transporting frozen items and things that should stay cold. Milk inside a hot car trunk will go bad in less than an hour.

Clean Cooking

Let's get back to cleaning everything. Start by cleaning the fresh fruits and vegetables. This is getting to be increasingly important, as recent outbreaks of illness from spinach and green onions have shown.[52] Getting most of these foods clean is easy—just rinse them thoroughly under cold running water. That includes fruits and veggies that are going to be peeled or that have thick rinds, such as melons. You don't need to use any sort of soap or bleach. These foods need to be clean, not sterile. Besides, eating soap or bleach isn't exactly good for you. If you're really concerned, there are nontoxic sprays that are designed for cleaning produce.

Unfortunately, there's one food that just can't be rinsed clean: raw sprouts. Bean sprouts, alfalfa sprouts, radish sprouts, and all the rest can be a real health risk, especially to children and people who have weakened immune systems. Best advice? Cook them. Never eat them raw.

Fresh-squeezed fruit or vegetable juices also can carry dangerous bacteria. Almost all commercial juice products are pasteurized—meaning they've gone through a safe heat process to kill germs—and packed into sterile containers, but some products aren't. Outbreaks of salmonella have been traced to unpasteurized juice from local cider mills and some unpasteurized organic products. You also could accidentally pass along germs when you make juice at home. Even pasteurized juices should always be stored in the refrigerated section of the store.

The bacteria found on meat, poultry, and seafood are killed by cooking. There's no need to rinse these foods first (and it would be hard to rinse ground beef anyway). What's far more important is to cook these foods thoroughly to be sure all the germs really do get killed. That means you can still have rare steak, because bacteria can't get into the center of a solid piece of meat—unless, of course, you use a fork to turn or move the steak. By stabbing it, you could force surface bacteria deep into the center of the meat. Use tongs instead.

Conversely, you should never eat a rare hamburger. The grinding process means that bacteria could be anywhere in the patty. When cooking a burger, the internal temperature needs to reach 160°F. Use a meat thermometer to be sure—a thick burger will turn brown and look done on the outside, but the inside could still be pink and not hot enough.

You can avoid just about any form of food poisoning by remembering a basic rule: keep hot foods hot and cold foods cold. When food sits out at room temperature, germs can get in and multiply. The two-hour rule applies here: if a food that should be hot or cold has been at room temperature for more than two hours, don't eat it. That applies to take-out food, too. Many a case of food poisoning has occurred when take-out food sat in a warm car or on a kitchen counter beyond the two-hour time limit.

My children used to try to tell me that whenever they dropped something edible on the floor, the five-second rule applied: it's OK to eat it if you pick it up in five seconds or less. I hate to shatter a child's illusions, but that's just not true. Even five *milliseconds* on a contaminated surface is enough for a cookie to pick up some salmonella or other bacteria. Remember how filthy floors are. People walk outside, step in bird and dog droppings, and transport these contaminants inside. It takes less than 15 or 20 bacteria to cause some forms of salmonellosis or *E. coli* infection. (To give you an idea how small that is, a couple hundred thousand bacteria can fit on the period at the end of this sentence.) The five-second rule really means, "Take five seconds to drop the food into the trashcan." Yes, there are people who go to bed hungry at night. But eating a poisoned cookie won't help them. Instead, be more careful in the future.

What's the germiest place in your house, according to the CDC? If you guessed the toilet bowl, you're right. That was too easy, though. What's the second-germiest place? It's your kitchen drain. That might be a bit of a surprise. And the third germiest? Your kitchen sponge.[53] That might be a big surprise, since you're always putting soap on it. Even so, germs love to lurk there—it's nice and moist, and there are tiny bits of trapped food to feed on. The other place they love to lurk is in cloth dishtowels. In either case, the germs get passed on whenever you wipe down a counter or dry your hands. To keep sponges and similar items clean, run them through the dishwasher or wash them in hot water and soap. And replace them often. Use paper towels instead of cloth for drying your hands, and wash cloth towels in hot water as soon as they get dirty.

Safe and Healthy Schools

Schoolchildren get sick with colds so often—and pass them on to you so often—that you probably figure it's inevitable. Well, children do get sick a lot, and sometimes it is inevitable, but not always. The best way to keep schoolchildren, their parents, and everyone else at school healthy is, of course, lots of handwashing. A few other tips:

- Send your children to school with disinfecting wipes to wipe down desktops and computer keyboards.
- Be sure your children carry tissue packets with them. Remind them to throw used tissues away quickly.
- Give children their own boxes of crayons. Sharing crayons among little hands spreads germs quickly.
- Try to keep shared toys clean. That's an almost impossible job, of course, but you can make a dent in it by washing stuffed animals often and wiping down other toys with disinfectant wipes.
- Be careful with backpacks—they're germ magnets. Children take their backpacks with them everywhere, including into the bathroom, where they drop them on the floor. Encourage children to hang their backpacks on the hooks in the bathroom and to keep them off the floor in other places. And don't let children dump their backpacks on their beds or the kitchen table when they get home! Wash the packs often.
- Use mechanical pencils. This sounds a little extreme, but it turns out that the dirtiest thing in a classroom is often the communal pencil sharpener.

Hygiene at Work

My work is being an orthodontist, so I'm surrounded by hygiene nuts at my office. Dental hygienists and dental assistants are the cleanest people you will ever meet. Our yearly expenditure for soap, hand sanitizers, and disinfectants exceeds the gross national product of many small countries. My staff and I are always washing our hands and sanitizing the treatment areas, the bathrooms, the reception room, and everywhere else—except my personal office. Sure, the carpet was vacuumed and the trash was emptied, but the office cleaners didn't touch my desk. That's because I had told them not to—I didn't want my papers getting mixed up. What that meant was that all the disinfecting that went on elsewhere never made it to my desk.

When I realized that, I started doing a little research. One study showed that the average office desk has 400 times more bacteria than the average toilet seat. [54]I was not happy to learn that I would be better off working at a toilet for a couple of hours a day than at my own desk.

Based on my research, I started using disinfecting wipes on my desktop a few times a day. I also started using them on the phone, the computer keyboard, and the computer mouse. My staff does the same. Are we healthier? I think so. Overall, my staff members take fewer sick days than they used to. But then again, they may just love their work!

CHAPTER 3

Eat Right

When it comes to proper nutrition, many folks are totally lost. They can't see the forest for the trees, and often concentrate on the wrong things. Yes, trans fats are bad. Yes, artificial ingredients should be avoided or limited. Yes, pesticides and hormones can make it into the food supply. Yes, your diet may be too low in certain vitamins or minerals. These are all serious problems of the American diet that should be addressed.

But the damage these ingredients do to your health is small compared to the damage that the real problems cause. The *major* problem with the typical American diet is one of excess: too many calories, too much fat, too much sugar, and too much salt. If you really want to improve your health, first concentrate on these Foul Four!

The First of the Foul Four: Too Many Calories

The largest health problem in America today is obesity. We eat too much and we are too fat. Between 20 and 30 percent of Americans are obese. Obese! Not just overweight, but actually obese! This epidemic of obesity is linked to early deaths from heart disease, diabetes, cancer, and infections. A 2008 study published in the *American Journal of Clinical Nutrition* shows that weight gain also is associated with systemic inflammation.[55] In chapter 1, we discussed how inflammation is linked to hardening of the arteries, high blood pressure, and heart attacks.

The saddest part about our obesity epidemic is that it doesn't have to be this way. Obesity is preventable.

Why do we overeat?

Obesity is caused by overeating—taking in too many calories for the amount of energy we expend. Why do we take in too many calories? It's not simply that we're hungry. Obesity is far more complicated than that. Conditions in America are perfect for practically forcing us into overconsumption. Our obesity epidemic is caused by a "perfect storm" of events.

A perfect storm refers to the simultaneous occurrence of events that, taken individually, would be far less powerful than the result of their chance combination. The perfect storm of obesity overtaking our nation is caused chiefly by the combination of five events peculiar to modern America.

1. Increased availability of food

During the history of mankind, there has always been a shortage of food. Indeed, evolution itself is largely driven by competition for food. Limited food supply in the ocean led primitive fish to venture onto land to sample land-borne berries and insects. The same problem in the African plains led giraffes to develop longer and longer necks to reach higher and higher for available leaves. Birds and reptiles evolved with different beaks specialized for different food sources so they could win the food competition.

Primitive humans' food supply was sparse and unreliable. There were long periods of drought, freeze, and famine. There was terrific competition for food, and many perished because they could not store enough calories during the good times to survive during the bad times. Thus, those early men and women whose genes were programmed to store extra energy as fat had a competitive advantage. The people who had "fat genes" who were good at storing fat survived. Those who had "skinny genes" often did not.

Today, some people joke that if they look at a cookie, their thighs get fatter. They are simply part of the majority. They are descendants of those survivors who had fat genes, programmed to store fat in preparation for the upcoming famine!

Fat genes work wonderfully during times of scarcity, famine, and starvation. However, they are a disadvantage in modern America. For the first time in history, there is an overabundance of food. Inexpensive food is available everywhere. It's in your face constantly. You can't avoid it. We've got *McDonald's* and buffets, *Twinkies* and chips, *Coke* and cappuccino.

This theory—that increased availability of food leads to increased obesity—was tested by University of Pennsylvania researchers in 2008. They used the U.S. Economic Census to examine the impact of the availability of fast-food restaurants on the weight of people who lived nearby in 544 counties in the United States. The researchers found that areas with the highest density of fast-food restaurants had the highest rates of obesity.[56]

All animals, including humans, are programmed to eat. It's in our hard wiring. We see food, we eat food. Thus, for the first time in human or animal history, with the overavailability of food, we eat and overeat. And then we eat just a little more.

2. Increased convenience

OK, so there's a lot of food out there. But if it weren't so darn convenient, we wouldn't overeat so much. You probably have an almost unlimited supply of flour, sugar, eggs, butter, and oil. But when was the last time you made yourself a doughnut? How is it then that 10 billion doughnuts were consumed in America last year? The answer is that it was convenient. You probably pass a doughnut shop a couple of times a day. There might even be one at the same place you fill your car with gasoline. It's just so easy, so convenient, to purchase and consume doughnuts today. That's why doughnut consumption has increase a million-fold over the past 50 years.

When I was kid, making popcorn was a major family event. We would get the bottle of oil out of the cupboard, pour it into a frying pan, and heat it up. In a separate saucepan, we would carefully melt the butter. We would open the can of popping corn, pour it into the frying pan, cover it, and vigorously shake until the popping was complete. My mom would dump the popcorn into a serving bowl, drizzle it with the melted butter, and we would attack! After the fun, we had to clean the frying pan, cover, saucepan, and bowl. We would dry the cooking utensils and put everything back in the cabinet. It was a lot of work, but even so, it was a special adventure to look forward to on Sunday nights.

Today, my children casually toss a bag into the microwave, set the timer to "popcorn," and two minutes later, they open the bag and devour the 200 calories inside. It's so easy that sometimes they repeat the procedure before their stomach has time to yell, "I'm full!"

You've got ice cream cartons in the freezer, cookie boxes in the pantry, cake on the counter, and wrapped candy everywhere. What could be easier than to overindulge?

3. Increased variety

The more varied your choice of food, the more you'll eat. It's that simple. Ask anybody who has been on a cruise. People on cruises tend to gain half pound a day due to the availability and variety of food. If it weren't for the variety, they would quickly become bored and stop eating (or at least slow down). People tend to try more, nibble more, and eat more as the variety increases.

If you wanted to, tonight you could dine on: beef or veal or pork or chicken or turkey or pasta or duck or lamb or tofu or apple or pomegranate or cake or cookies or ice cream or banana or tuna or lobster or crab or bass or trout or reconstituted soy protein. You have a wider choice of food for dinner tonight than did either Caesar or Napoleon! If a multimillionaire living in New York City in 1920 wanted a pepperoni pizza at nine o'clock at night, he would have to wake his chef, then wait for the ovens to heat, the dough to rise, the sauce to cook.

Today you live better than that millionaire did. You just pick up the phone, and the pizza is delivered 30 minutes later. How lucky are you? But watch yourself. All this variety may lead to overeating.

4. Television

People who watch a lot of TV take in more calories than people who watch less TV.

That's pretty simple and straightforward. You watch, you eat. You have your favorite shows; you have your favorite snacks. Dozens of studies have shown that people develop TV-watching-and-eating routines. They mindlessly consume ice cream during dramas and chips during sports.

This mindless eating habit, which often develops during childhood, can easily add 500 to 1,000 calories per day to your diet!

5. Lack of exercise

Here's where the obesity "perfect storm" really gets rough! Not only do we eat too much because of availability, variety, convenience, and TV watching—we've also stopped exercising! You don't burn many calories while driving, watching TV, sitting at a computer, or eating. You burn calories when you exercise, and exercise we don't.

There are two basic forms of exercise: purposeful and non-purposeful. Purposeful exercise is exercise for exercise's sake: running, swimming, aerobic dancing, weight training, using a treadmill or rowing machine. But modern Americans are too busy doing all the other stuff they do to allow time for purposeful exercise. With a 90-minute round-trip commute, 8-hour work day, 2.8 hours of television, 1.2 hours of internet surfing, parenting, eating, socializing, shopping, bill paying, and grooming, who has time to exercise?

And non-purposeful exercise … where did that go? Washing machines, dishwashers, automobiles, elevators, escalators, indoor shopping malls, and just plain exhaustion and laziness have all but removed non-purposeful exercise from our way of life.

At this point you may be surprised that, given the perfect storm, the obesity rate is only 20 or 30 percent. Well, folks, it ain't over yet! Keep watching the statistics. The childhood obesity rate is the highest ever, and obese children tend to become obese adults. Chances are the obesity rate will continue to skyrocket for the next several years.

Calories in, calories out

What is a calorie, anyway? It's a unit of energy. One calorie is the amount of heat it takes to raise the temperature of one gram of water by one degree Celsius. So, let's say you were to burn a chocolate chip cookie in a well-equipped laboratory. You'd discover that the cookie gives off about 50,000 calories in heat—which seems like way more than would be possible. Actually, it isn't. When nutritionists talk about the calories in food, they make the big numbers easier to deal with by giving them in kilocalories. There are 1,000 calories in a kilocalorie, so a nutritionist would say the cookie has 50 kilocalories. In everyday usage and in food labels, though, the "kilo" gets dropped and we just talk about the calories.

The important thing is that calories are an accurate way to measure the amount of energy contained in each gram of what we eat and drink. The more calories in a food, the more energy it contains. Remember, though, that just because a food is high in calories and therefore high in energy, that doesn't mean it's good for you. Potato chips, for instance, are high in calories, but it's hard to make a good argument for them as a healthy food choice.

The food and beverages we consume are made up of three basic calorie-containing components: carbohydrates (starches and sugars), protein, and fat. One gram of carbohydrate or protein contains 4 calories. One gram of fat contains 9 calories.

To determine how many calories you need each day, you need to look at your energy balance—the calories you consume versus the calories you expend. Or, more simply: "calories in, calories out."

To maintain your current weight, the calories you take in from food and beverages needs to equal the calories you burn as part of your normal metabolism, your regular daily activities, and any extra physical activity. To gain one extra pound of weight, you have to take in approximately 3,500 more calories than you expend. To lose one extra pound of weight, you have to expend approximately 3,500 more calories than you consume. Again, to put it more simply: take in fewer calories, and/or burn more calories, and you'll lose weight. Take in more calories and/or burn fewer, and you'll gain.

The problem is that it's very easy to get your energy balance out of whack. Two factors come into play. The first is your age. We need fewer calories as we get older, but not many of us want to admit we're getting older, especially if it means having to watch what we eat. The second factor is activity. The more sedentary you are, the fewer calories you need.

Exactly how many fewer calories? Here's how it breaks out:

Calories by Sex, Age, Activity Level

		Activity Level		
Women	**Age**	**Sedentary**	**Moderately Active**	**Active**
	19–30	2,000	2,000–2,200	2,400
	31–50	1,800	2,000	2,200
	51+	1,600	1,800	2,000–2,200
Men	19–30	2,400	2,400–2,600	3,000
	31–50	2,200	2,400–2,600	2,800–3,000
	51+	2,000	2,200–2,400	2,400–2,800

Source: National Institutes of Health

As you can see from the chart, the difference between a good energy balance and one that will make you pack on the pounds isn't that great. If you're a 55-year-old woman who is moderately active, you need about 1,800 calories a day. If you eat 2,000 calories a day—just 200 extra calories—without also increasing your activity level, you'll gain a pound in about three weeks. And all it takes to gain that extra pound would be four extra 50-calorie chocolate chip cookies every day. The flip side of that, though, is that by cutting your daily calories by 200, you'd lose a pound in about three weeks—faster if you also increase your activity level. That doesn't sound like much, but a pound every three weeks or so works out to about 17 pounds over the course of a year.

How much is enough?

Yet another reason for today's soaring rates of overweight and obesity is that we've lost track of healthy portion sizes. It's all too easy to take in a lot more calories than you need without even realizing it. As just one example, here's the calorie count for a typical meal at *McDonald's*:

- *Big Mac* sandwich: 540 calories
- Large fries (6 ounces): 570 calories
- Baked apple pie: 270 calories
- Medium *Coke* (21 fluid ounces): 210 calories

The total calories add up to 1,590—and that's just lunch. Even if you had a diet drink and skipped dessert, you're still at 1,110 calories. And if you went in the opposite direction and had a medium chocolate milkshake instead of the *Coke*, that would add an amazing 770 calories. Think the chicken nuggets are better for you? Not really. A 10-piece serving is still 420 calories.

As goes *McDonald's*, so goes every fast-food restaurant—and every other type of restaurant as well. Ditto for the portion sizes of everything else, from frozen pizza to soft drinks. It's all too easy to take in far more calories than you realize.

Size matters

The typical serving of a food today has become so large that it's hard to know exactly what a healthy portion really is. The "Nutrition Facts" label on every food package is supposed to help you figure that out. It does, sort of. But you need a good understanding of nutrition, the ability to do some mental math, and a healthy dose of skepticism for the label to be helpful

For example, look at the nutrition facts on a package of chocolate chip cookies. The information on the label is based on the health issues that the Food and Drug Administration (FDA) and the U.S. Department of Agriculture (USDA), in their combined wisdom, consider to be of greatest concern to the general public. That information starts with the serving size. For each serving, the label lists total calories, calories from fat, total fat, saturated fat, trans fat, cholesterol, sodium, total carbohydrates, dietary fiber, sugars, protein, vitamin A, vitamin C, calcium, and iron. That's a lot of information. Let's break it down.

The serving size is the first piece of information at the top of the label. This information is both helpful and misleading. The serving size is usually given as a standard kitchen measurement—½ cup, for instance—followed in parentheses by the equivalent amount in grams. If the food is eaten by the piece, the serving size is given that way instead—three cookies, for instance.

The serving information is accurate, down to the last gram. What can make it misleading is that the serving size is almost always smaller than the amount you're probably going to eat. Half a cup of almost anything is a pretty small serving. And will you really stop at just three small cookies? Everything else on the label is based on that small serving size, though, which makes it all too easy to underestimate how much you're eating.

Fortunately, the information on the next line lets you get a better handle on serving size by telling you how many servings per container are in the package. If the serving size is ½ cup and the package contains four servings, you can "eyeball" your portion by taking out one-quarter of the amount in the container.

Next on the label is the amount of calories per serving. This can be misleading, too. Let's say one serving—three small chocolate chip cookies—is 150 calories. Well, you think to yourself, that's not so bad—just 50 calories a cookie.

True, 50 calories for a single cookie isn't bad by itself. But 150 calories for three cookies starts to add up. And once again, will you really stop at three small cookies? And, of course, what about eating those three cookies as dessert after eating your *Big Mac* and large fries?

One thing you have to remember about the real world is this: food doesn't just disappear! It really doesn't. That piece of cake on the counter that keeps getting smaller and smaller? Somebody is eating it! And it may be you! A little bit here and a little bit there sure adds up. Cake doesn't disappear, and the calories don't disappear either.

But, let's say you decide that you're normal weight and are pretty active, so you can easily afford the 150 calories from those three cookies. From a strictly caloric approach, you can; but from a nutritional approach, you can't. Here's why: next on the nutrition list are the total fat and cholesterol counts for the food. Indented below the total fat count is a breakdown of the types of fats. In the case of those chocolate chip cookies, the fat is likely to be mostly saturated fat—the undesirable kind. And if the food contains saturated fat from animal sources, it also will contain cholesterol. As I'll explain later in this chapter, dietary fat and cholesterol are necessary for good nutrition, but most of us get much more than we need. Extra saturated fat and cholesterol from high-calorie, low-nutrition foods is not the ideal way to get these nutrients.

The Second of the Foul Four: Too Much Sugar

Name something a baby loves: candy! Name something Americans love: candy!

Sugar! We love it! Each American eats, on average, 153 pounds of it per year. It's hidden in almost everything, from ketchup to canned soups, from luncheon meat to salad dressing. It's in soft drinks and mixed drinks, juices and apple sauce.

Sugar causes cavities and periodontal disease. It's also linked to obesity, diabetes, cancer, osteoporosis, and cardiovascular disease. It's cheap and tastes good, but it is nothing but empty calories. It contains zero vitamins, minerals, or fiber. Furthermore, sugar has long been used as a preservative in jellies and jams because in high amounts it's toxic to bacteria! It kills them, and in the long run it can make you ill, too.

Sugar is just one form of carbohydrate. Carbohydrates are starchy or sugary foods that have a similar molecular structure. But there are subtle differences in the structures of different carbohydrates, and these structural differences cause major biochemical differences when we eat these foods.

The building blocks of *all* carbohydrates are sugars. There are several different kinds of sugars, but the most common sugars in carbohydrates are glucose and fructose. All of these are small, sweet-tasting molecules made up of six carbon atoms plus oxygen and hydrogen atoms (hence the name Carb-O-Hy-drate).

As you may have surmised, apples, oranges, bananas and other fruits are sweet because they are high in fructose. So is—as the name implies—high-fructose corn syrup, a processed food made from, well, corn!

Table sugar, or the common sugar you buy for baking or cooking, is sucrose. Sucrose is actually made up of two sugar molecules: one molecule of glucose holding hands with one molecule of fructose. Sucrose, like the single molecule sugars glucose and fructose, is considered a *simple carbohydrate.*

The second type of carbohydrate is the *complex carbohydrate* called starch. Starch is a long molecule, made up of dozens or hundreds of glucose molecules holding hands. Because the molecule is so long, it does not have a sweet taste. Bread, potatoes, pasta, and rice all contain a lot of starch.

A third type of carbohydrate is the complex carbohydrate called cellulose. Cellulose, like starch, is also a long molecule. But the glucose molecules in cellulose hold hands much tighter than they do in starch. In fact, the molecules hold hands so tightly that your body can't separate the glucose molecules. Cellulose can't be digested, so it actually passes right through you. Fiber is made of cellulose. So are the stems and leaves of most vegetables. Believe it or not, wood and paper also are cellulose.

Most grains, fruits, and vegetables are high in cellulose and/or starch. They also tend to be high in other nutrients, such as vitamins, minerals, and antioxidants. However, during the refining process, food manufacturers can remove the majority of these nutrients. What's left is refined carbohydrates.

Good carbs and bad carbs

Carbohydrates are often misunderstood. The confusion over carbohydrates comes in part from the popularity of weight-loss diets like *Atkins* and *South Beach* that sharply limit your intake of carbohydrates. The diets give the impression that all carbs are bad; but in fact, once you get past the most restrictive initial stage, what these diets do is eliminate bad carbs and moderately limit your intake of good carbs.

That brings us to the difference between bad carbs and good carbs. As more and nutritionists agree, it's an important distinction, not just for weight loss but for overall good health.

Bad carbs are carbohydrates that have been so heavily processed that the natural nutrients in them have been largely stripped away. Enriched white flour is a good example. To make it, the bran, or inner husk, of each grain of wheat is stripped away. With the bran goes the B vitamins, iron, and fiber. The germ (the part of the grain that contains the embryo of a new plant) is also stripped away—there goes the vitamin E. What's left is so low in nutrients that the government makes flour producers add some vitamins back, which is why it's called "enriched" flour.

Sugar and foods that are high in sugar or high-fructose corn syrup also are major bad carbs. This includes cookies, cakes, candy, doughnuts, soft drinks, and a whole lot of other foods as well.

Bad carbs are high in calories and low in nutrition. That's bad enough, but here's what's worse: because they're low in fiber, and because your body absorbs processed carbohydrates quickly, eating a lot of bad carbs doesn't make you feel satisfied. Think of eating six chocolate chip cookies in a row. It's all too easy to do that and still want more. Now think of eating six apples in a row. Almost impossible, right? Between the water and fiber in the apples, and the work it takes to chomp through them, you'd be full quickly—and you'd stay full longer.

The difference in calories and carb grams is substantial. A single medium chocolate chip cookie contains about 100 calories, 7 grams of bad carbs, and 0 grams of fiber. A single apple contains about 80 calories, 21 grams of good carbs, and 3 grams of fiber—and no dietary fat. So, eat all six cookies, and it'll cost you at least 600 calories and around 42 grams of bad carbs. Force yourself to eat three apples, and you get just 240 calories, 63 grams of good carbs, and 9 grams of fiber, plus 160 mg of potassium and 0 mg of sodium. In addition, the apples make you feel full longer, so you're less likely to snack on other foods or overeat at your next meal.

A diet high in processed carbs is likely to make you gain weight, but the damage could be even worse than just extra pounds. When you eat these foods, the carbohydrates in them are digested and converted to blood sugar quickly. Very quickly! That means they hit your system with a lot of blood sugar all at once, which puts a real strain on your body's ability to handle it. If you already have high blood sugar problems from prediabetes or diabetes, bad carbs can make your blood sugar spike up and stay up. That's not good. Even worse, that spike might be followed by a crash as your body overcompensates and sends your blood sugar plummeting.

Good carbs are high-carbohydrate foods that have been minimally processed so that the nutrients and fiber are still there, and little or no sugar or fats have been added. Fruits, starchy vegetables, and whole grains—such as whole wheat, barley, oatmeal, brown rice, and corn—are all good carbs that are high in natural fiber and nutrition. When you eat these foods, the fiber in them slows down the digestive process. Instead of causing your blood sugar to spike, these foods are converted to blood sugar more slowly and steadily.

It's easy to change to your diet to decrease bad carbs and increase good carbs. Swap a serving of french fries for a baked potato, for instance. By choosing the baked potato and being sure to eat the delicious skin, you get the fiber and nutrients that are in the potato along with the carbohydrates, and you ensure those carbs will enter your system evenly instead of in a rush. Compare that to a serving of french fries: No fiber, few vitamins, extra fat from the deep-frying oil, usually along with lots of extra salt and perhaps some sugary ketchup. To make the difference really stand out, take a look at this chart:

	Large Baked Potato	**20 French Fries**
Calories	281	334
Carbohydrates	63 grams	40 grams
Fiber	6 grams	3 grams
Sodium	21 mg	614 mg
Potassium	1,627 mg	540 mg
Vitamin C	38 mg	3 mg

Even though you get fewer carbohydrates from the french fries, you get more calories, less fiber, a lot more sodium, a lot less potassium, and practically no vitamin C. Add a tablespoon of ketchup to those fries and you add 16 calories, 4 grams of carbs, and another 178 grams of sodium. The healthy choice is pretty clear.

There are plenty of other simple choices you can make to trade good carbs for bad. As a general rule of thumb, whole-grain foods should make up at least half your daily intake of grains. In other words, make *half* your daily grains *whole*. Read the labels carefully—whole grain should be the first ingredient. Swapping white bread for whole wheat or multigrain bread is easy to do. Whole-wheat pasta is another easy swap.

Breakfast is a great place to start your good-carb day. In our home, we always have an open box of all-fiber cereal on the counter. My children will mix the all-fiber with their favorite cereal for a tasty yet nutritionally sound breakfast. And never sprinkle sugar on your food!

Trading candy, cookies, cake, doughnuts, and other high-carb foods for better choices is more difficult. Foods that are naturally sweet, such as fruit, are still a lot less sweet than cookies, and they don't have that succulent feel in your mouth that comes from added fat. And let's face it: sometimes you just need to have some chocolate!

You don't have to give up the occasional sweet treat or completely deprive yourself of chocolate. Once you start trading in the processed foods for more natural ones, though, you may find that cookies, doughnuts, and other processed foods suddenly seem almost sickeningly sweet. And once your taste buds get used to the rich flavors of naturally sweet, unprocessed foods, prepared foods seem to taste more of their chemical additives than their main ingredients.

To get away from foods with added sugars, check the ingredients label. If sugar or high-fructose corn syrup is listed as one of the first few ingredients, stay away.

What about sugar-free foods? As a dentist, of course, I recommend sugar-free chewing gum, candy, and soft drinks. As for other sugar-free foods, however, be cautious. Manufacturers often make up for the missing sugar by adding more low-quality carbohydrates. In the end, you end up with just as many calories, bad carbs, and fat.

Eat your veggies

One really good way to lower your intake of bad carbohydrates, calories, and dietary fat is to eat more fresh fruits and vegetables. Instead of more french fries, choose more broccoli and some extra salad. Instead of more cheese puffs, more baby carrots. Instead of apple pie, apples. It's pretty simple, really.

Today's dietary recommendations call for five or more servings of fruits and veggies every day. Amazingly, few Americans manage to do this. Most of us manage only two or three a day, which goes a long way in explaining why so many of us are overweight. Five or more servings a day sounds like a lot, but isn't really all that hard to do. That's because a serving is actually a fairly small amount—usually four ounces, or about one-half to one cup.

What does that work out to? For leafy greens and salad greens, four ounces is about a cup; for other veggies, about half a cup cooked. That would be only five broccoli florets, or half of a large bell pepper, or six baby carrots. For fruit, it's one medium piece, or four ounces of 100 percent fruit juice. For smaller fruits, a serving might be four large strawberries, or sixteen grapes, or a medium wedge of cantaloupe.

Looking at how small the portions are, you can see how simple it would be to add just one extra portion a day. Once you've gotten used to that, it's simple to add another extra portion. Give it a few months, and you'll easily be up to five or more servings every day.

The Third of the Foul Four: Too Much Salt

You can't live with it. You can't live without it.

Our ancient ancestors evolved from the sea, where salt is plentiful. On land, far away from our primordial beginnings, salt is an important part of our physiology. Salt is absolutely essential for our survival. It is used in nerve transmission, muscle activity, food absorption, and energy and water balance. Salt, or its components, are part of the membranes of each and every human cell.

You are programmed to desire salt. Along with sweet, bitter, and sour, salt is one of the four basic tastes that your tongue can distinguish. Salt brings out flavor in foods, and it was one of the first food additives. The ancients cherished it because not only is it tasty and necessary for life, but it was the first food preservative, used thousands of years before refrigeration or artificial preservatives. Even dogs love it, and that's why they'll lick your face and hands in search of the salt left over from evaporated sweat! Years ago, when salt was at a premium, something valuable was "worth its weight in salt."

Today, salt is cheap and omnipresent. It's in everything. The average American consumes about 4 grams (4,000 mg) of salt per day. That's about twice the recommended amount.

Salt is known chemically as sodium chloride. Nutritionists use the two terms more or less interchangeably, and on nutrition facts labels, salt is listed as sodium. Generally, the more salt you eat, the higher your blood pressure will be—and high blood pressure is not a good thing for your health. When your blood pressure is high, your risk of heart attack, stroke, congestive heart failure, and kidney disease is high, too.

Some people are simply more sensitive to the blood pressure effects of salt than others. You may not be able to tell if you're salt-sensitive, but the likelihood is greater if you fit certain categories:

- You've already been diagnosed with high blood pressure.
- You're of African-American descent. High blood pressure is more common among people with African ancestry.
- You're older than age 50. Salt sensitivity increases with age.

If you have any of these characteristics, most doctors recommend keeping your salt intake on the low side. The recommended maximum amount is no more than 2,300 mg a day. However, if you have—or if you're at risk for—high blood pressure, keeping your daily sodium at half that or less is a good idea.

A high intake of salt also may lead to atrophic gastritis. This condition causes the stomach lining to waste away, and can lead to stomach cancer. This means that a high-salt diet can increase the risk of stomach cancer even in people who are not salt-sensitive.

It's not that hard to reduce your salt intake. We get most of our excess salt from prepared and packaged foods, and from salty snack foods. I hope by now you realize that you can easily do without the empty calories and extra salt from potato chips, pretzels, cheese puffs, and all the other snack foods. It's hard to get away from the convenience of prepared and packaged foods, though. To cut your salt intake from these products, look for lower-sodium versions where possible. This doesn't necessarily mean choosing a reduced-sodium or low-salt product. There's a surprising range of salt content in similar products. For example, the amount of sodium per serving in similar prepared salad dressings can vary by several hundred mg! By comparing labels of different brands, you can still enjoy your favorite type of dressing— just chose the brand with the least salt. The same holds true for many other foods, including canned soup, frozen vegetables, frozen pizza, even bread and pretzels. Also check labels for phrases such as "low in sodium," "no added salt," and "very low sodium."

Salt is only half the story when it comes to high blood pressure. Cutting back on salt definitely helps, but what's just as important is increasing your potassium intake. Potassium works along with sodium to correctly balance the amount of water in your cells and in your blood. If the balance gets out of whack, your body tends to hold onto too much fluid, which raises your blood pressure. A good way to get the balance out of whack is to eat a diet that's high in salt and low in potassium. And that's easy to do, because the best dietary sources of potassium are fresh fruits and vegetables, and most of us don't eat near enough of these. At the same time, we eat too many processed and snack foods that are high in salt. A good balance of potassium and salt is roughly five parts potassium to one part salt, but the typical American actually gets one part potassium to two parts sodium—or twice as much salt as potassium. Is it any surprise that roughly 30 percent of all American adults have high blood pressure? Or that among people older than age 65, more than half have high blood pressure?

Lowering your sodium intake and raising your potassium intake is a good idea even if you don't already have high blood pressure. A 1997 study in the *Lancet*, a renowned British medical journal, showed that older adults who lowered their salt intake also sharply lowered their risk of stroke—even if they didn't have high blood pressure.[57]

Further proof of how more potassium and less sodium helps your health comes from the ongoing research of the Dietary Approaches to Stop Hypertension (DASH) study. Participants in the 1997 DASH study and its 2000 follow-up were divided into two groups. One group ate the typical American diet; the other ate a low-fat diet that was much higher in fruits and vegetables. Both groups ate about 3,000 mg of salt every day. However, the typical-diet eaters took in only about 1,700 mg daily of potassium, while those who ate high amounts of fruits and vegetables—naturally good sources of potassium—got about 4,700 mg of daily potassium. Guess whose blood pressure went down? You're right: the fruit-and-vegetable group members saw their readings drop, while the typical-dieters' readings stayed the same or went up. What's very interesting about the study is that among the fruit-and-vegetable eaters, the people who had the highest blood pressure experienced the largest drop.

There's hardly a more compelling argument for eating more fruits and veggies and fewer potato chips. Good dietary sources of potassium include leafy greens, such as spinach and collards; carrots; potatoes; bananas; citrus fruits; berries; kiwis; and grapes.

The Final Part of the Foul Four: Too Much Fat

Even as Americans are getting heavier all the time, their fear of eating fat is getting worse. While it is true that Americans generally eat too much fat, you do need dietary fat to live—and some types of fat are actually good for you.

Your body needs fat for energy; to carry fat-soluble vitamins such as vitamins A, D, E, and K to your cells; and to make cell membranes and hormones, among other important functions. The USDA's dietary guidelines recommend getting between 20 and 35 percent of your daily calories from fats. Most people, however, get a lot more than that; typically, 35 to 40 percent of their daily calories come from fat.

So is it all that fat that's making us fat? Yes and no. A gram of fat has 9 calories, while a gram of carbohydrate or protein has only 4. On the other hand, fat slows down digestion and sometimes makes us feel full faster and longer. This might help to control overeating—except that most of us eat so quickly, we pack the calories in far faster then the signals can reach our brain to tell us we're full.

If you're not careful, you might cut back on fats but end up eating more bad carbs and getting the same number of calories—or maybe even more. It's the *SnackWells* Syndrome. When *SnackWells'* low-fat cookie was introduced in the early 1990s, it was a real hit. Consumers snapped them up, confusing low-fat with low-calorie. In fact, *Snack-Wells* had almost as many calories as regular cookies. To make the cookies taste good, the manufacturer had simply replaced the bad fat with bad carbs, particularly more sugar. Snacking on *SnackWells* didn't magically help people lose weight, even though the cookies were indeed lower in fat. (When the low-carb fad was at its height, low-carb cookies were popular, which just goes to prove that every dietary fad has its own cookie.)

Even so, it's easy to overdo the fats. That's because they're everywhere, especially in foods that already have a lot of calories: chocolate bars, french fries, processed foods, ice cream, cheese, and of course, nice, juicy steaks.

The problem isn't just that fat makes us fatter. It's that some fats make us not only fatter but sicker. Saturated fat and trans fat are the culprits behind diseases such as diabetes, heart disease, certain cancers, and maybe even Alzheimer's disease.

Dietary fat falls into three categories: good, bad, and terrible.

The **good fats** are unsaturated fats. Without going into a long explanation, these are fats, such as vegetable oil, that are liquid at room temperature. They're good because they provide you with the nutrition you need without clogging your arteries. The good fats fall into three basic types:

- Monounsaturated fatty acids: found in nuts and seeds and vegetable oils, especially canola oil, olive oil, and sunflower oil
- Polyunsaturated omega-6 fatty acids: found in vegetable oils, especially soybean oil, corn oil, and safflower oil
- Polyunsaturated omega-3 fatty acids: found in walnuts; flaxseed; oily fish, such as salmon and tuna; and vegetable oils, especially soybean oil and canola oil. Omega-3 fatty acids also are available as supplements, usually in the form of fish oil and/or flaxseed oil capsules.

The **bad fats** are saturated fats. These are fats, such as butter and lard, that are solid at room temperature. Saturated fats are found mostly in animal foods, such as meat, poultry, eggs, milk, and other dairy products. Animal foods also contain cholesterol, a fatty substance that is a building block for fats. If you eat a lot of saturated fat and cholesterol, you may raise your own level of LDL cholesterol—that's the bad kind, the one that's implicated in clogged arteries and heart disease.

The **terrible fats** are trans fats. These are also known as partially hydrogenated vegetable oils—unsaturated vegetable oils that have been heavily processed to be solid at room temperature. Trans fats are widely used in processed foods—especially baked goods, such as cookies, crackers, cakes, and snack foods—and in french fries. It's also used in some stick margarines and solid shortenings. Trans fats are so artificial that your body can't metabolize them well. What that means is that trans fats not only raise your LDL (bad) cholesterol, they also actually lower your HDL (good) cholesterol.

Here's what the famed *New England Journal of Medicine* said about trans fats in a major article in 1999: "Metabolic and epidemiological studies indicate an adverse effect of trans fatty acids on the risk of coronary heart disease. Furthermore, on a per-gram basis, the adverse effect of trans fatty acids appears to be stronger than that of saturated fatty acids."[58]

Let me translate: this stuff is really bad for you.

Because trans fats are so terrible, food manufacturers are trying to cut back on them. Even so, there are still lots of foods with trans fats out there. It's another excellent reason to cut back on heavily processed foods in your diet.

OK, what's the bottom line here? How much of what kind of fat should you eat?

- Overall, limit your total dietary fat intake to between 20 and 35 percent (preferably on the low end) of your total calories.
- Limit saturated fats to no more than 10 percent of your total calories.
- Choose unsaturated fats from fish, vegetable oils, and nuts whenever possible.
- Don't eat trans fats.

To put all that into practical terms, figure that if you eat 2,000 calories a day, no more than 700 of those calories, and preferably fewer, should come from fat of any kind. And of those 700 calories, no more than 70 should come from saturated fat. To put that in fat grams, if you eat 2,000 calories a day, your fat intake should be between 45 and 75 grams a day. Of that total, no more than 20 grams should be saturated fat.

There are plenty of easy ways to cut back on saturated fat in your diet. One of the simplest is to switch to low-fat dairy products, such as low-fat yogurt and cheese. You'll save fat grams—and calories, too. One ounce of regular cheddar cheese, for instance, has 6 grams of saturated fat and 114 calories. The low-fat version has 1 gram of saturated fat and only 50 calories.

Strong Bones and Your Diet

Low-fat dairy products have another important advantage: they're a good dietary source of calcium and vitamin D. You need both nutrients to build and maintain strong bones throughout your life. Think of it this way: your bones need plenty of calcium and vitamin D to build up their thickness and strength as you grow, a process that continues until you're about 30. After that, the natural aging process means you start to drawn down your bone account, whether you're a man or a woman; but for a woman, the natural bone loss that comes with aging can really accelerate after menopause. That's when a woman no longer produces estrogen, which plays an important part in maintaining bone density. Too much bone loss can lead to osteoporosis.

Getting plenty of calcium and vitamin D in your diet can help prevent osteoporosis as you get older, but the most important time for these nutrients is when you're younger and your bones are still thickening. Soda and other soft drinks, however, shove milk out of the diet, especially among teens and young adults; so do worries about the calories and fat in dairy products. The result is that many young people today just aren't getting enough calcium and vitamin D to build bones that will stay strong for a lifetime. In fact, USDA studies show that nearly 90 percent of American women aren't getting the recommended 1,200 mg of calcium each day.

Low-fat dairy is a good solution to this problem, because the amount of calcium stays the same even as the fat gets taken out. One 8-ounce glass of nonfat milk, for instance, has about 300 mg of calcium, or about a quarter of your daily recommended intake. Cheese is another good source; 1 ounce of low-fat American cheese has 124 mg of calcium. There are over 400 mg of calcium in 8 ounces of low-fat yogurt.

Vitamin D works synergistically with calcium to help build and maintain strong bones. Your body produces vitamin D in a complex process that starts with sunshine on your skin. Milk has added vitamin D, while eggs and organ meats are natural dietary sources. Unfortunately, just as we're all afraid to eat dietary fat these days, we're also all afraid to get any sunshine. We're constantly being warned to put on sunscreen (with good reason) on those rare occasions when we venture away from our televisions and computers and actually go outdoors. The result is that many people, from children all the way up to the elderly, are low on vitamin D. Here, too, low-fat dairy products can help, but getting outdoors every day also is important.

A 2008 study by the Institute for Cancer Research in Oslo showed that the health benefits from the sun outweigh the risk of skin cancer.[59] Modest sun exposure gives enormous vitamin D benefits, which help the immune system to fight against internal cancers such as colon cancer, lung cancer, breast, and prostate cancer.

So use common sense. Enjoy the sunshine, and be reasonable with your use of sunscreen lotion.

Weighing in on Calories

About two-thirds of all adult Americans now weigh too much. They're at least 10 pounds heavier than the upper range of a healthy weight for their height. To find out where you stand, you need to know your body mass index (BMI). This is the modern replacement for older height/weight charts. The calculations used are a little more accurate, but the basic idea is the same. The BMI chart looks at your height and gives you a range of weights, going from underweight all the way up to seriously obese. Each step is numbered and covers a range of about 5 to 10 pounds. The normal BMI range is 19 to 24. If your BMI is 25 to 29, you're overweight; if it's 30 and above, you're obese. Because the BMI charts include a range of weights for height, you no longer have to decide if you have a heavy or light build as you did with the older charts. The drawback to the BMI charts is that you can't tell yourself you're not fat, you just have big bones—the ranges take care of that. If you're a woman who's five feet six, for instance, the range of normal weight is from 118 to 148 pounds. That means you could be on the skinny side of normal at 118 pounds, or near the overweight end of normal at 148 pounds—a 30-pound range.

The formula for figuring out your BMI is: 703 times your weight in pounds divided by your height in inches squared. It's a lot simpler to just look it up in the chart on the following page.

So, check the chart to see if your BMI is within the healthy-weight range of 19 to 24. If your BMI is less than that, you probably need to gain weight; if it's greater than that, you probably need to lose some weight.

But even if you're within the normal range, you may not be eating a healthy diet. If you're like most Americans, chances are you're not eating enough fruits, vegetables, and whole grains—only about 20 percent of us do. Chances also are good that you're eating too many highly processed and sugar-laden carbohydrates, and getting too much of the unhealthy dietary fats and not enough of the good ones.

Another factor here is your waist size. Are you an apple or a pear? You're an apple if you carry extra fat in your belly area. You're a pear if you carry extra fat in the buttocks and legs. For reasons that aren't entirely clear, apple-shaped people are more vulnerable to heart disease, diabetes, and high blood pressure, even if they're at a healthy weight. To find out if you're at risk, use a tape measure to measure your waist size just above your hip bones (without clothes). No matter what your weight or height, a healthy waist size is less than 40 inches for men, and less than 35 inches for women.

Activity Level and Calorie Intake

Once you've figured out a healthy weight for you, the next thing to look at is your usual level of physical activity. That's your typical amount of daily exercise, leaving out the occasional weekend-warrior activities. You need to have a good handle on this to determine how many calories you need to maintain or achieve a healthy weight, so be honest with yourself here. Look at how much physical activity you do, on average, every day, and decide which category best fits you:

- Sedentary. You only do light physical activity as part of every-

Body Mass Index Table

	Normal						Overweight					Obese										Extreme Obesity															
BMI	19	20	21	22	23	24	25	26	27	28	29	30	31	32	33	34	35	36	37	38	39	40	41	42	43	44	45	46	47	48	49	50	51	52	53	54
Height (inches)																Body Weight (pounds)																				
58	91	96	100	105	110	115	119	124	129	134	138	143	148	153	158	162	167	172	177	181	186	191	196	201	205	210	215	220	224	229	234	239	244	248	253	258
59	94	99	104	109	114	119	124	128	133	138	143	148	153	158	163	168	173	178	183	188	193	198	203	208	212	217	222	227	232	237	242	247	252	257	262	267
60	97	102	107	112	118	123	128	133	138	143	148	153	158	163	168	174	179	184	189	194	199	204	209	215	220	225	230	235	240	245	250	255	261	266	271	276
61	100	106	111	116	122	127	132	137	143	148	153	158	164	169	174	180	185	190	195	201	206	211	217	222	227	232	238	243	248	254	259	264	269	275	280	285
62	104	109	115	120	126	131	136	142	147	153	158	164	169	175	180	186	191	196	202	207	213	218	224	229	235	240	246	251	256	262	267	273	278	284	289	295
63	107	113	118	124	130	135	141	146	152	158	163	169	175	180	186	191	197	203	208	214	220	225	231	237	242	248	254	259	265	270	278	282	287	293	299	304
64	110	116	122	128	134	140	145	151	157	163	169	174	180	186	192	197	204	209	215	221	227	232	238	244	250	256	262	267	273	279	285	291	296	302	308	314
65	114	120	126	132	138	144	150	156	162	168	174	180	186	192	198	204	210	216	222	228	234	240	246	252	258	264	270	276	282	288	294	300	306	312	318	324
66	118	124	130	136	142	148	155	161	167	173	179	186	192	198	204	210	216	223	229	235	241	247	253	260	266	272	278	284	291	297	303	309	315	322	328	334
67	121	127	134	140	146	153	159	166	172	178	185	191	198	204	211	217	223	230	236	242	249	255	261	268	274	280	287	293	299	306	312	319	325	331	338	344
68	125	131	138	144	151	158	164	171	177	184	190	197	203	210	216	223	230	236	243	249	256	262	269	276	282	289	295	302	308	315	322	328	335	341	348	354
69	128	135	142	149	155	162	169	176	182	189	196	203	209	216	223	230	236	243	250	257	263	270	277	284	291	297	304	311	318	324	331	338	345	351	358	365
70	132	139	146	153	160	167	174	181	188	195	202	209	216	222	229	236	243	250	257	264	271	278	285	292	299	306	313	320	327	334	341	348	355	362	369	376
71	136	143	150	157	165	172	179	186	193	200	208	215	222	229	236	243	250	257	265	272	279	286	293	301	308	315	322	329	338	343	351	358	365	372	379	386
72	140	147	154	162	169	177	184	191	199	206	213	221	228	235	242	250	258	265	272	279	287	294	302	309	316	324	331	338	346	353	361	368	375	383	390	397
73	144	151	159	166	174	182	189	197	204	212	219	227	235	242	250	257	265	272	280	288	295	302	310	318	325	333	340	348	355	363	371	378	386	393	401	408
74	148	155	163	171	179	186	194	202	210	218	225	233	241	249	256	264	272	280	287	295	303	311	319	326	334	342	350	358	365	373	381	389	396	404	412	420
75	152	160	168	176	184	192	200	208	216	224	232	240	248	256	264	272	279	287	295	303	311	319	327	335	343	351	359	367	375	383	391	399	407	415	423	431
76	156	164	172	180	189	197	205	213	221	230	238	246	254	263	271	279	287	295	304	312	320	328	336	344	353	361	369	377	385	394	402	410	418	426	435	443

Source: Adapted from *Clinical Guidelines on the Identification, Evaluation, and Treatment of Overweight and Obesity in Adults: The Evidence Report.*

day life. You don't have a job that's physically active, and you don't deliberately add any activity to your life.

- Moderately active. In addition to the light physical activity of daily living, you add in some daily activity, roughly the equivalent of walking a mile or two at a moderate pace.
- Active. In addition to the light physical activity of daily living, you add in activity roughly equivalent to walking three or more miles a day at a moderate pace.

As a general rule, the more active you are, the better. For most people, being physically active is more important than being at a normal weight. (In fact, exercise is so important that I've devoted an entire chapter to it later in this book.) It's probably better to be fit and fat—to have what's sometimes called "hard fat"—than to be of normal weight and unfit. Overall, of course, it's best to be both fit and of normal weight.

Is Organic Really Healthier?

Organic foods are a major source of confusion about healthy eating. Most organic foods are a lot more expensive than their conventional alternatives. Are they really so much better for you? Are they worth the extra money?

Like so much else in nutrition, it all depends.

Let's start with the definition of organic. Back in 2002, the USDA released a new set of standards that define organic food products, and provided a federally approved organic seal that can be used on food labels. According to the new standard, the organic label can be used on foods that are produced without using conventional pesticides, petroleum-based fertilizers, sewage-sludge fertilizers, genetic engineering, or irradiation. Organic meat, poultry, eggs, and dairy products come from animals that are given no antibiotics or growth hormones.

The USDA has a strict inspection process for organic foods. In fact, it's so strict and takes so much paperwork that a lot of small local farmers can't comply—even though they use organic or sustainable methods. But on the other hand, a 100 percent organic food grown thousands of miles away on a huge corporate farm and then transported to your local supermarket has a big environmental footprint—and it isn't all that fresh by the time it reaches you. A local grower may not be able to do all the work to get the USDA label, but his product is farm-fresh and has far less environmental impact. Also, many local farmers are certified as organic growers by local organizations or state agencies, even if they don't have federal certification.

Because organic foods are produced without artificial fertilizers, pesticides, and other chemical additives, eating them reduces your exposure to toxic substances that could harm your health. And, organic foods are often—though not always—more flavorful than their conventionally produced counterparts. If foods are locally grown, they're often fresher and tastier. Studies show that many organically grown foods also are higher in minerals and vitamins.

Supporting organic farming goes beyond health and taste, however. By buying these products, you are helping to reduce the overall use of chemical fertilizers and pesticides, which, in turn, protects the environment. By buying organically produced milk, meat, poultry, and eggs, you help reduce the agricultural use of antibiotics and hormones, and encourage humane farm management. Organic farming doesn't create toxic runoff that pollutes water and disrupts ecosystems, and it helps preserve and improve farm soil.

All to the good, and good reasons to buy organic foods. But organic foods are usually more expensive compared to their conventional alternatives. (A friend of mine refers to one organic supermarket chain as "Whole Paycheck.") Not only that, but the selection is limited. Do you really need to buy organic for good health? Yes for some foods, no for others.

On the "yes" list are foods that are the most likely to contain harmful pesticide residue. Not too surprisingly, these foods also are the most likely to be produced by the sort of industrial agriculture that causes a lot of environmental harm. Buying the organic version limits your exposure to harmful chemicals.

I strongly recommend buying the organic versions of these foods: milk, peanut butter, apples, bell peppers, celery, cherries, grapes, lettuce, nectarines, pears, potatoes, spinach, and strawberries.

It's probably not worth the added expense for these foods: asparagus, avocadoes, bananas, broccoli, cabbage, corn, kiwis, mangoes, onions, papayas, peas, and pineapple. These have little pesticide residue.

What about everything else, like, say, cucumbers or carrots? Well, if a pesticide kills bugs, it's probably not too good for you, either, so I recommend choosing the organic product whenever possible.

When organic isn't available, you can still limit your exposure to chemical residue if you rinse all produce under running water; remove the peel from fruits and vegetables; and take off the outer leaves of leafy vegetables, such as lettuce or kale.

When you're trying to buy organic foods, don't be fooled by other labels. Food manufacturers throw around the word "natural," for example, but it doesn't really mean anything. There are other labels that don't have a standard definition, aren't regulated, and aren't verified by an independent third party, and don't mean the same thing as "organic." These include the following claims: "antibiotic-free," "hormone-free," "free-range," "free-roaming," and "cage-free."

Bottom Line

You can eat a low-fat, low-salt, all-organic diet and still be overweight, sedentary, and unhealthy. There's no magic bullet here—no special food that will miraculously make the pounds melt away and muscles grow. And avoiding some foods won't magically keep you slim and healthy, either. What's needed are common sense and moderation.

Of course, that's easy to say, but a lot harder to do. Diets are notoriously hard to stick to, and firm resolutions to work out more are broken all the time. I've found that the most effective way to lose weight and shape up is to make small, gradual changes. It's not a diet or exercise program, it's a lifestyle choice: you're deciding to live a healthier life, feel better, and reduce your risk of chronic disease.

CHAPTER 4

Think Right

The most important thing you can do to assure a happy, healthy life is to maintain a positive attitude! You've probably heard this a million times, but just like washing your hands and brushing your teeth, this advice is tried and true—and invaluable. It's something we all know we should do, but few of us actually strive to do it. Too frequently we fall back into our old habits of anger, despair, fear, and helplessness.

Maintaining a positive attitude isn't easy; otherwise, we would all embrace this lifestyle. Like exercise and weight control, it demands self-control. Like most things in life, it becomes easier with practice.

You may be thinking, "Will just being positive really make a difference?" If you believe that you're getting a raise, will it actually *get* you that raise? If you believe that your family will be safe, will that *keep* them safe? If you believe that your plane will take off on time and land safely, will that belief assure that your trip will go as planned? If you believe that you can beat cancer, will it really improve your chance of survival?

The answer is yes. And no.

Wishful thinking alone can't accomplish much. Wishful thinking is fine for children, but it's just a beginning when it comes to developing a positive attitude. A positive attitude goes far beyond mere wishful thinking. A true positive attitude requires determination, consistency, and willpower. A positive attitude requires that you change the way you filter the world around you.

Let's take one example from the scenarios above. Will just believing that your plane will take off on time and land safely ensure a smooth trip? No, wishful thinking won't help here. But a positive attitude sure will! Here's how:

First, choose your flight wisely. Early flights generally are more predictable, and they give you far more leeway in the event of a problem. Next, plan on arriving at the airport early. That way you won't be so stressed as you wait in the lines for boarding passes and security. I always tell my family that I'd rather arrive at the airport two hours *before* the plane takes off rather than two minutes *after* the plane took off!

If the plane is delayed, enjoy yourself instead of complaining. Read, take a stroll through the concourse, get a bite to eat, or just relax. Complaining or worrying won't help at all, but it will make you feel bad. Instead, accept that this is the way of the world, and make the most of it. Understand this: You are at the airport. Your flight is delayed. There is nothing you can do about it. Now decide. The choice is yours: do you want to be miserable, stressed out, and depressed? Do you want to complain to your fellow travelers? Or do you want to have a positive attitude and make the most of your situation? Either way, you will be late. Which do you want to be? Do you want to be content or miserable? The decision is entirely up to you—not the airline, not the airport, and not the situation.

Also understand that if you are late, no matter what happens, you can handle it! Remain positive. You know you can handle it because you've handled situations like this before. If you're late for the meeting, you can handle it! If you miss the event, you can handle it! Somehow, you can and *will* handle it, so feeling anxious or depressed that the plane is late is simply not an option.

Once you're in the air, relax and understand that you're safe. There should be no "fear of flying." The facts are that flying is safe. Airplanes almost never, ever crash. Every day tens of thousands of planes take off and land, and there's never an accident. By the end of every week, hundreds of thousands of planes have taken off and landed without incident. By the end of each year, *millions* of planes have done the same. There's so much more evidence and reason for positivism then negativism. You must train yourself to see this and maintain a positive attitude. (We'll talk about ways to do that a little later in this chapter.)

Many successful people—politicians, philosophers, industrialists, and others—know that while you can't always control your situation, you can always control your attitude. Positive thinking is absolutely necessary for happiness and success. Here's a sampling of insights from some well-known achievers:

Happiness does not depend on outward things, but on the way we see them.
—*Leo Tolstoy (1828–1910)*

Most folks are about as happy as they make their minds up to be.
—*Abraham Lincoln (1809–1865)*

You can't control the wind, but you can adjust the sail.
—*Bill Anderson (1937– present)*

The world is good-natured to people who are good-natured.
—*William Makepeace Thackeray (1811–1863)*

Happiness doesn't depend upon who you are or what you have. It depends solely upon what you think.
—*Dale Carnegie (1888–1955)*

The greater part of happiness or misery depends on our dispositions, not our circumstances.
—*Martha Washington (1731–1802)*

Always bear in mind that your own resolution to succeed is more important than any one thing.
—*Abraham Lincoln (1809–1865)*

Self-confidence is the first requisite to great undertakings.
—*Samuel Johnson (1709–1784)*

Formulate and stamp indelibly on your mind a mental picture of yourself as succeeding. Hold this picture tenaciously. Never permit it to fade. Your mind will seek to develop the picture.
—*Norman Vincent Peale (1898–1993)*

The real secret to success is enthusiasm.
—*Walter Chrysler (1875–1940)*

Whether you think you can or whether you think you can't, you're right!
—*Henry Ford (1863–1947)*

Opportunity is missed by most people because it is dressed in overalls and looks like work.
—*Thomas Edison (1847–1931)*

The greatest discovery of my generation is that a human being can alter his life by altering his attitudes of mind.
—*William James (1842–1910)*

I have been through some terrible things in my life, some of which actually happened.
—*Mark Twain (1835–1910)*

Our attitudes make the difference between happiness and misery. So why do we allow a negative attitude to destroy our lives? Here's the answer: We *use* our attitude to *judge* our attitude, so it always seems OK. No matter how much misery and failure our attitude may cause, we always defend our attitude! We rationalize our bad attitude with justifications. Think of the cranky old man who lives down the street. He's always complaining that the children make too much noise, or that you're parking on "his side of the street." You know the type. Everybody thinks he's a cranky old man—except him. He feels that his feelings are justified. He justifies his bad attitude, as we often do for ourselves.

Imagine this scenario: a woman finishes reading this book and decides she's always going to maintain a positive attitude. But her alarm clock fails to go off, she gets up late, and her teenage daughter is fresh to her during breakfast. She snaps back at her daughter because *she believes this time she really has a right to do so.* Because of the traffic, she arrives at the airport late. Because of the earlier fight with her daughter, she forgot her cell phone. Now her attitude begins to slip, and she feels justified. It's not her fault. She feels that she has a right to have a bad attitude—her daughter caused it. The woman finally gets on the plane, and after it sits for an hour on the runway, she blows up at the flight attendant. (*It's not my fault. It's the fault of all these incompetent idiots. I have a right to be angry! I have a right to be annoyed! Now everything is going wrong!*) Her bad attitude did not help her situation one iota. She is still late, but now she also is miserable and unhappy.

Your Two Brains

You have two brains—really. One brain sits on top of the other. Your lower brain, sometimes referred to as your "reptilian brain," controls most of your behavior as well as the feelings we call "attitude." The lower brain does not use language. Your other brain, called the cerebral cortex, sits on top of the lower brain. Your cerebral cortex is responsible for language and logic. Your two brains act independently, but they're "wired" together.

The behaviors in the lower brain aren't in words, so they can't be translated by your upper brain. Instead, your upper brain is forced to deduce reasonable rationalizations to make sense of the behaviors it observes.

The connection between the two brains is imprecise. Normally, you don't think about, nor are you aware of, the body systems and activities controlled by your lower brain: breathing, eating, swallowing, walking, even throwing and catching a ball. Similarly, your attitude or mood is normally controlled by your lower brain. You are happy, sad, positive, or negative without thinking about it.

The fact that behaviors are normally controlled by the lower brain doesn't mean that the upper brain can't have significant input. Just as athletes can practice and improve their throwing and catching skills, constant practice can improve your skill at controlling your attitude.

Your upper brain sends out a constant stream of messages. These messages can keep you up late at night, or cause you to laugh at inappropriate times. These messages can make the difference between a positive attitude and a negative attitude.

A positive attitude, in and of itself, is great. It makes you happier. It makes you enjoy life more. It helps you to achieve success. But by no means does it guarantee success. You must also include diligence and hard work.

Accentuate the Positive

One of my favorite stories when I was a kid was *The Little Engine that Could*. You remember that one: it's about the little steam engine that keeps telling himself, "I think I can, I think I can," until finally he actually does succeed in pulling the train over the mountain. After he succeeds, he congratulates himself by saying, "I thought I could, I thought I could." I've always had a positive outlook on life, and I'm sure reading that book often when I was young has something to do with that. When my own children were little, I used to tell the story to them, and I think it helped them grow into the positive young people they are today.

Just like the Little Engine, our cerebral cortex sends a stream of thoughts through our minds, so constantly and so fast that we don't really notice. Psychologists call this inner monologue "self-talk." I call it your "verbal chatterbox." If your self-talk is made up of mostly negative messages, it will program your lower brain to have a pessimistic outlook on life.

Let's say you've got a big deadline at work and you're falling behind. If your self-talk is negative, you'll be saying to yourself, "I can't believe how stupid I've been about this. I should have started on this weeks ago. I would have if I hadn't had so much other work to do. Now I'm going to have work late every night and all weekend. The boss is going to kill me if I miss this deadline." This is typical negative self-talk: full of self-blame, complaining, distortion, and expecting the worst. And, it only makes the situation worse by raising your stress level and making it even more likely that you'll miss your deadline.

What if you turned all those negative statements into positive self-talk? You could say to yourself, "OK, I could have started this a little sooner, but I had to get some other important work out of the way first. I know I can work efficiently and get this done on time, even if it means staying late a couple of times. And the boss will be impressed that I made my deadline." Your positive self-talk helps you see the situation realistically, make a positive plan to get the work done, and anticipate a positive result. You calm down; take a positive, optimistic approach; and you get the work done—just like the Little Engine.

Changing your negative self-talk isn't all that hard, but you do have to make a conscious effort. Whenever you find yourself making negative statements, stop and think about how to turn them into positives instead. For example, every time you think to yourself, "I'll never get any better at this," try thinking, "I know I can master this." Instead of, "I can't figure this out," try, "I'll look at this from another angle." Instead of, "This is too complicated," try, "I'll take this step by step so I won't feel overwhelmed." Swap the negative words in your vocabulary for positives. Change every "can't" to a "can," every "won't" to a "will."

Self-talk doesn't change instantly from negative to positive, but if you work at it consistently, your negative messages will gradually become more positive and realistic. It takes a lot of practice, not unlike the athlete trying to perfect a batting swing or golf putt. But the work will pay off: you'll have a more positive approach to life and feel more in control.

Affirmations

One way to learn what positive self-talk really sounds like is to use affirmations. An affirmation is a short, simple, positive statement of fact or belief that you repeat to yourself. For example, if you're worried about giving a talk to your colleagues, try repeating the affirmation, "I'm a good speaker." By expressing this to yourself, you turn a negative, limiting belief—that you're not a good speaker—into a positive belief.

Affirmations work because what we say to ourselves often becomes a self-fulfilling prophecy. If you consciously repeat positive affirmations to yourself, your unconscious mind starts to believe them and work toward them. And striving toward positive goals is always more fun and less stressful than being upset.

Affirmations seem to work best if they're short, simple, positive, and in the present tense. That's exactly what I did many years ago when I was speaking at a health fair sponsored by a large department store chain. It was important for me to really rock the audience! So I prepared well. I did diligent research about the topic and the audience. I prepared stories and practiced my gesticulations. And I kept telling myself over and over again, "They're going to love me! It's going to be great! I am going to be spectacular!"

It worked. I actually received a standing ovation. But understand, it wasn't just my positive attitude. (That would have been wishful thinking.) It was my positive attitude *combined with* my hard work! I accomplished what I set out to do—and so can you!

It all comes down to this: if you think positively, you'll act positively. You'll be healthier, happier, and more fulfilled by your life. What could be simpler?

Positive Attitude Traps

Be careful not to fall for the common "positive attitude traps." These traps may create a temporary positive attitude, but you'll quickly rebound into even worse negativity.

- Drugs. Both illegal and prescription medications can become crutches. They might make you feel good for a little while … but at what price?
- Food. Thirty percent of Americans are obese. We're clearly not eating all that food because we're hungry. We're eating it to feel good. But the short-term pleasure gained from overeating simply adds to depression and poor attitude in the long run, when we feel uncomfortable in our clothing and in our mirrors.
- Shopping. OK, shopping fuels our economy, and we all want the latest gadgets and fashions. But is all that shopping making us happy?

America is by far the most prosperous, affluent civilization the world has ever seen. We have larger homes and more stuff than anyone else. However, we are far, far from the happiest civilization. According to the National Institute of Mental Health, in any given one-year period, 9.5 percent of the population, or about 20.9 million American adults, suffer from a depressive illness. Acquiring more possessions won't make you feel better over time, won't satisfy you, and won't contribute to a positive attitude. You will only want still more possessions as soon as you tire of your most recent treasure.

I'm not saying that you should give up all your worldly possessions and renounce materialism. Certainly not! Simply understand that we are often manipulated by advertisers to buy expensive products that, in the long run, won't make us happy or contribute to a positive attitude.

Keep in mind how lucky you are to have your sight, rather than just a new LCD TV. Imagine how many people would trade their deafness for that new iPod you want to buy. With this type of thinking, it's far easier to maintain a positive attitude!

Attitudes and Stress

A positive attitude also goes a long way toward combating stress. And when it comes to stress, we need all the help we can get.

You probably already know that stress can cause health problems or make existing problems worse. Conversely, reducing stress by learning how to manage it can play an important role in preventing illness and improving your overall health. But this is one area where common sense can be hard to apply. You may know that working overtime for too many days on end is highly stressful and bad for you, but you also might feel there's not much you can do about it—which only adds to your stress! In reality, there *are* steps you can take to lower your stress level, even when life seems to be piling the stress on faster than you can handle.

What Is Stress?

Stress is one of those words that gets thrown around so much that it has lost some of its real meaning. The word is now loosely used to mean anything from a mild annoyance to a major traumatic event. From a medical and psychological perspective, however, stress has a specific meaning. We define stress as a change that causes physical, emotional, or psychological strain. Stress usually means something bad, but not every change is negative. Even positive changes can be stressful, as anyone who has ever planned a wedding knows. In fact, positive stress—for example, working hard to complete a challenging project in an area that really interests you—often can be enjoyable.

Negative stress is much more of a problem because over the long run, negative stress can have serious health consequences. Generally speaking, negative stress falls into two broad categories: acute and chronic.

Acute stress happens all at once: you have a close call while driving, for instance, or you have a brief confrontation with someone. Your heart pounds and your blood pressure may rise, but when the incident is over, your body returns to normal and you put it behind you. (There are some people whose lives seem to be nothing but one episode of acute stress after another. We usually call these people "teenagers.")

Chronic stress is stress that is ongoing and inescapable. It could be from a job you hate, a bad relationship, or the demands of caring for someone who's ill. In fact, it could be from simply trying to juggle family life, work, and all the other demands of modern living. Any situation that makes never-ending demands over a long time will cause chronic stress. This is the sort of stress that causes physical and psychological problems, and can even lead to premature death.

There's one other type of stress that's important to understand: post-traumatic stress disorder, also known as PTSD. People with PTSD have generally experienced a frightening or dangerous event, such as rape, assault, combat, a serious car crash, and the like. Symptoms of PTSD are usually severe, and include problems such as serious depression, sleep disorders, nightmares, flashbacks, inability to form relationships, and anger issues. PTSD is more common than most of us realize, and people who suffer from it often don't get the understanding and help they need. It's a serious condition—too serious to discuss here. If you or someone you know is suffering from PTSD, please seek professional help.

Chronic Stress

Your body reacts to an episode of acute stress by triggering your natural "fight-or-flight" response. In earlier times, when you were threatened by a saber-toothed tiger, you had to make a snap decision: should I attack the tiger with my spear, or run away from it as fast as I can? To help you throw the spear harder or run faster, your body released hormones, especially the stress hormones known as catecholamines. The best-known stress hormone is epinephrine (also called adrenaline). It's the epinephrine that sped up your heart rate, slowed your digestion, increased the blood flow to your arms and legs, and overall gave you a burst of energy and strength. If you also were lucky, you survived to hunt another day.

In the days when you had to worry about encountering saber-toothed tigers, the fight-or-flight response was crucial to your survival. The response was employed only occasionally, when it was really needed. Today's world is less dangerous, but your body doesn't know that. You still get the same surge of hormones whenever you find yourself in a stressful situation, such as being stuck in a long line at the motor vehicle office. The situation is far from life-threatening, but your body still responds as if it were.

Fortunately, when it comes to acute stress, your body also knows that when the danger is past—the tiger has run away or the clerk has finally called your name—it's time to stop making stress hormones and return to normal functioning. This is known as the relaxation response, and for most people, it starts to happen soon after the stressful moment has passed.

But what if the stress never really goes away? What if you are exposed to multiple physical and emotional stressors every day of your life? Your body never gets to stop making stress hormones, and the relaxation response never really gets to kick in. When your body is constantly exposed to elevated levels of stress hormones, bad things start to happen.

Chronic Stress and Your Health

Chronic stress has been linked to a long list of health problems, either as a primary cause or as a factor that makes a condition worse. Depression, diabetes, heart disease, obesity, periodontal disease, and possibly cancer all are related to chronic stress. So are sleep disorders, frequent headaches, migraines, and muscle and lower back pain. Chronic stress also damages your immune system and makes you more likely to get sick with infections such as a cold or the flu. Chronic stress can even affect your reproductive organs, causing painful menstrual periods, decreased fertility, loss of desire, and erectile dysfunction.

And that's just the physical symptoms. On the emotional side, chronic stress can lead to anxiety, depression, lack of energy, irritability, difficulty concentrating, and poor attitude.

Your heart is one of the first organs to be damaged by chronic stress. Stress makes your body need more oxygen, which makes your heart pump faster. At the same time, stress raises your blood pressure, which makes your heart work harder to get your blood to circulate. At first, chronic stress might cause you to have an elevated heart rate and high blood pressure. If it continues, you might develop shortness of breath, chest pain, and abnormal heart rhythms. And all that, in turn, can lead to a heart attack, heart failure, stroke, or even sudden death from an arrhythmia. Several solid studies have directly linked heart attacks and high levels of chronic stress—especially when the stress comes from your work. A recent study in the *Journal of the American Medical Association* points to an increased risk of a second heart attack among people who experience chronic job stress.[60] Any sort of chronic stress, however, can have a long-term impact on your heart health.

Your immune system also can be affected by chronic stress. Long-term exposure to cortisol, one of the major stress hormones, has been shown to weaken immunity and make people more susceptible to illness. You've probably noticed that you're more likely to catch a cold when you've been under a lot of stress. Excess cortisol is part of the reason. The other part is probably that when we're under a lot of stress, we can't make good lifestyle choices, such as eating well and getting enough sleep.

Stress also is one of the most common triggers of headaches. In fact, mild headaches are often called tension headaches. Stress and tension make us tense up the muscles of our shoulders, neck, and scalp. That reduces blood flow to the muscles of the head, causing the headache. Serious headaches, or migraines, can be triggered by hormonal changes that are caused by emotional stress, such as anxiety or depression. For both types of headaches, learning to manage stress can be a big help.

If you have diabetes, chronic stress is likely to make it worse. When your body releases stress hormones, they impact your production of insulin. That's the hormone that carries blood sugar into your cells. It's a complicated equation, but for most people, chronic stress raises blood sugar levels. If you also have diabetes, your blood sugar is already high, so chronic stress can make a bad situation worse. In fact, just having diabetes is stressful in itself! On top of that, if you're under a lot of stress, you may not be able to watch your diet and get enough exercise to keep your diabetes under control. And, stress might lead you to drink more alcohol than usual, which also can raise your blood sugar.

What about chronic stress and cancer? The evidence here is less clear. We know that the immune system is a major defense against cancer. And, we know that stress can make the immune system less effective. But there's conflicting evidence to link stress-induced changes in the immune system to cancer. The confusion is illustrated by studies of breast cancer. Some recent studies of women with breast cancer have shown significantly higher rates of the disease among women who had a traumatic life event or loss, such as the death of a husband, within several years of their diagnosis. On the other hand, a 1996 study of self-reported stress among women with breast cancer showed little connection between stressful life events and breast cancer risk.

Researchers also have been looking at how stress can affect the outcome for women who already have breast cancer. One well-known 1989 study showed that women who participated in a support group—which presumably helped reduce the stress of having breast cancer—lived longer than those who didn't.[61] But follow-up studies since then haven't always borne this out. Additional studies of people diagnosed with other types of cancer also have shown that emotional well being has little influence on cancer survival; positive thinking and an optimistic outlook don't always prolong life.

What the breast cancer studies *have* shown, however, is that women who participate in support groups have less stress and an overall better quality of life, which is certainly desirable. Interestingly, exercise—which, as I'll discuss a little later in this chapter, is helpful for reducing stress—also seems to improve quality of life for women who have breast cancer, and may improve survival rates as well. Several good studies have shown a similar effect for gentle yoga.

In a good example of how chronic stress can affect not only your health but the health of those around you, a recent study looked at the stress experienced by the daughters of women who have breast cancer. The study suggests that this stress may increase the daughters' risk of developing the disease themselves. Of course, the daughters are already at higher genetic risk, but the ongoing stress of coping with their mothers' condition can raise their levels of stress hormones. This, in turn, impairs their immune systems and leads to a reduction in the special immune cells that kill cancer cells. So far the evidence is just in the laboratory, but researchers are planning an intervention study that would teach stress-reduction techniques to these young women and track their health as they age.

The brain, too, is affected by chronic stress. When your stress response goes into overdrive for a long period, stress hormones continuously bombard your brain cells. Over time, that can actually change your brain circuitry and rearrange the neural networks that coordinate thought, emotions, and reactions. It's no surprise that high levels of stress are related to forgetfulness, inability to focus, reduced problem-solving skills, and irritability.

Stress and poor attitude also can cause chronic inflammation, a problem discussed at length in earlier chapters. The Air Force Health Study, published in 2007, showed a direct connection between emotional stress and high levels of chronic inflammation.

There's one other big health issue associated with chronic stress: substance abuse. If you're always under a lot of stress, you're more likely to do things your body doesn't like, such as smoke, drink too much alcohol, use drugs, and overeat.

Symptoms of Chronic Stress

People suffering from chronic stress may not even realize it's happening. And if you don't realize that you're under a lot of stress and you need to take some steps to reduce it, you've got a good chance of being headed for serious health problems. How can you tell that the stress is becoming too much for you? Look for these telltale symptoms:

- Sleeping problems. Are you sleeping too much or too little?
- Changes in eating habits. Are you gaining or losing weight?
- Low energy. Do you feel tired or without energy most of the time?
- Loss of interest. Do the things you used to enjoy no longer interest you?
- Mood changes. Are you easily irritated, angered, or saddened?
- Physical health. Are you getting a lot of headaches, upset stomachs, colds, or other health problems?

Did you answer yes to at least one question? If so, it's time to start looking into ways to reduce your stress. If you answered yes to more than one question, your stress level may be getting dangerously high.

Stress Reduction: Get to the Source

Unfortunately, chronic stress is pretty much a fact of life for most of us. Even when we love our jobs and have a happy family life, we all still have work-related and family-related stresses—to say nothing of all the other unavoidable stressful events of daily living. (Some people even think going to the dentist is stressful. I don't know why.)

Since we can't avoid stress—and let's face it, life would be boring without at least some stress—the next best thing is to learn ways to manage it so that it doesn't cause health problems or interfere with our enjoyment of life.

The first step in getting your stress under control is figuring out what's stressing you. A lot of the time, the cause is perfectly obvious because it involves a major life change. The change could be a good one—the birth of a child, for instance—or a negative one, such as a death in the family. Either way, big changes are stressful. As a general rule, life changes cause us to go through a period of high stress, and then we gradually adapt. After a while, the stress lessens and our life returns to a more normal pattern.

Perhaps the most stressful time of my life was when my dad died. He was not only my dad, he also was my partner. We met for breakfast every day at seven in the morning, and stayed with each other until six in the evening. His death was devastating to me.

For a while, my daily patterns and routines changed. I stopped exercising, and for a short period of time, I even stopped teaching. However, after the grieving period was over, my normal, positive attitude returned. I still miss my dad, and I value the times we had together; but the major stress of this life change has gradually resolved.

Other stresses are more likely to be ongoing. Job-related stress, for example, is extremely common. Many studies have shown that the less of a sense of control you have in your job, the more stressed you're likely to feel, no matter what your job is. In fact, if you have a lot of responsibility but not a lot of control over your work, you're more likely to have stress-related illnesses.[62]

Job stress can come from a lot of sources:

- Poor communication. If you and your boss or coworkers aren't communicating well, the resulting frustration and irritation can be a major source of stress. Poor workplace communication also can lead to a feeling that you lack support—an additional source of stress.
- Too much responsibility. When you feel overburdened with too much work, too much responsibility for other people and their work, or unrealistic deadlines, you're much more likely to feel stressed out.

- Lack of meaning. When work doesn't provide a sense of meaning or pride, it becomes stressful. This sort of stress is surprisingly common, even among high-level workers who seem to have fulfilling jobs. In reality, people can feel overwhelmed by their work, have doubts about their ability to do it well, or feel they're not being challenged enough.
- Insecurity. Worries about being laid off or fired, needless to say, are a major source of job stress. Poor self-esteem—feeling insecure about yourself and your abilities— also can cause chronic stress.

Health problems—your own or those of someone close to you—can be another major source of stress. Having a chronic disease, such as diabetes, severe arthritis, heart disease, cancer, or some other serious health problem, is difficult. Being a caretaker for someone else who has a serious health problem can be just as stressful. As our population ages and as people live longer with ongoing health problems, caregiver stress is becoming a more widespread problem. In fact, about one in four American families today care for someone over the age of 50. About 75 percent of caregivers are women; two-thirds of caregivers are holding down full-time jobs in addition to caring for someone. All those caregivers are under a lot of physical and emotional strain—and the stress can be very damaging. Caregivers are more likely to be depressed or anxious; studies suggest that they're also more likely to have health problems such as diabetes and heart disease.

Emotional problems, which are often linked to physical problems, also are a cause of stress. Feelings of depression, anxiety, grief, or anger cause stress. They also may be the other side of the stress coin. You might not be able to tell which factor is the cause and which is the effect, but the good news is that helping one usually helps the other.

Another significant cause of chronic stress is personal relationships. Going through a break-up, divorce, or period of strained family relationships is very stressful. So is having a chaotic or unhappy home life; but even a happy, busy family can be a source of stress if you feel overstretched or underappreciated (or both). The opposite problem of feeling alone in life can also cause significant stress. People who don't have close relationships or strong friendships are more likely to have chronic stress. People who do have a good network of social relationships, on the other hand, have been shown to live longer and to have less decline in function as they age.[63]

As you can see from all the above, there are a *lot* of ways to get totally stressed out! I've found that simply stopping long enough to think for a few minutes about what exactly is causing your stress is a good way to start reducing it. Simply identifying the source can give you some perspective, and it can help you realize that there are simple ways to get on top of your stress—instead of letting it get on top of you.

Stress Reduction Techniques

OK, you can't control everything in your life, and stress will inevitably creep in. How you handle it helps make the difference between feeling overwhelmed and feeling in control. And that can make the difference between bad decisions and good ones, between bad health and wellness. These simple stress-reduction techniques can help you feel more relaxed and better able to handle problems as they come up:

Exercise. Any form of exercise, even a short walk around the block, is a great way to reduce stress and improve your health at the same time. A daily walk of just 30 minutes or so is even better, not just for your mental health, but also for your heart health. Why? It's not just because the physical activity gives your heart and the rest of your body a mild workout; it's because exercise also lowers stress. It works because the physical activity helps to counteract some of the effects of the stress hormones. When you produce a lot of cortisol, for instance, it increases your resistance to insulin. This in turn means that your blood sugar can go up too high. Exercise improves insulin resistance and lowers your blood sugar.

Exercise also releases the brain's powerful chemical messengers, such as endorphins and dopamine. These brain chemicals have a lot to do with feeling optimistic and calm—the so-called "runner's high" is caused by them. Fortunately, endorphins and other messengers are released even through mild exercise, so you don't have to train for a marathon to feel the benefits.

Exercise also distracts you from the things that are causing stress in your life. It doesn't make those things go away, but getting a little distance from your problems helps you put them in perspective. Many people find that yoga, with its emphasis on both the body and the mind, is a great de-stressor—but any type of exercise will help. The important thing is find some a convenient form of exercise you like to do, and then do it regularly. Any sort of physical activity—even housework—helps. A regular workout keeps ordinary daily stress from building up, and also lets you work off any unusual stress.

Time for yourself. Often stress leaves us feeling overwhelmed by demands from others. We feel pulled in many directions at once. One of the best ways to counter this feeling is to make some personal time for yourself and do something that's meaningful and enjoyable to you. That could be sitting quietly and reading a book, listening to music, or working on a favorite hobby. It could also be something more active, such as taking an aerobics class or volunteering for the neighborhood cleanup. What's important isn't what the activity is; it's that you've chosen to do it for yourself.

Whenever I recommend this approach to people, I often hear "Oh, I'm too busy for that." I respond, "Exactly, which is why it's even more important." Making time for yourself might take a little juggling at first, but it pays off. Lowering your stress level makes you feel better and gives you more energy and focus. And that will help you be more productive so you can get through all the things that were keeping you so busy—and stressed—that you didn't have any time for yourself.

Progressive relaxation. To help you cope with the tight muscles, headaches, and overall feeling of tension that stress can cause, progressive relaxation can be a helpful technique. It's easy to learn:

1. Find someplace quiet where you can lie down for about 15 minutes: your bed, a couch, even the floor. Make yourself comfortable and close your eyes.

2. Starting at the top of your head, consciously relax your muscles. You'll be able to feel the tension leaving them.

3. Move down your body, consciously relaxing the muscles as you go. Relax from your head to your shoulders and chest, down your arms to your hands, and down your legs to your feet.

4. Lie quietly for a few minutes. If you have the time, start consciously relaxing again from the top.

Progressive relaxation can sometimes work a little too well. I learned to do progressive relaxation by taking a short class where the instructor talked us through it. At the end of 15 minutes, four out of the ten students were asleep! If you haven't been getting much sleep because stress has been keeping you up at night, this might not be a bad thing; but if you need to stay awake, try setting a timer.

Sometimes, such as at work, even 15 minutes of quiet and privacy can be hard to find. In that case, try a few minutes of deep-breathing instead:

1. Lie down if you can; if not, sitting in a chair is fine.

2. Rest your hands on your abdomen.

3. Inhale slowly and deeply through your nose to the count of four. You should be able to feel your abdomen rise.

4. Hold your breath for just a second or two. Then slowly breathe out again through your mouth, again to the count of four.

5.   Repeat five to ten times.

Visualization. In this technique, you sit quietly in a comfortable place. Then you imagine yourself in a calm and pleasant situation that's enjoyable for you—relaxing on a beautiful sunny beach, for instance. Go deeply into the scene, focusing on how it looks and feels. If you're imaging a beach, for instance, focus on the crash of the waves, or imagine the feel of the sand between your toes. By visualizing the relaxing situation, you actually do relax yourself. Think of it as a 10-minute mental vacation.

Another approach to visualization is to imagine yourself doing something successfully. This is a useful approach for reducing performance-related stress; it's used by many professional athletes. Since most of us aren't professional athletes, however, let's look at a more common situation. Let's say you have to give a speech and you're worried that it won't go well. Using visualization can help you handle the stress and give the speech with confidence.

Sit quietly in a relaxing place and imagine yourself giving the talk. Start at the beginning, as you're being introduced, and imagine every step, all the way to the part where you say, "Thank you very much for listening," and you step down from the podium. Focus on how well you will do it and how glad you will feel when you have succeeded. If you reach a point in the visualization where you start to feel anxious or can't clearly imagine what will happen, back up a bit and repeat that point until you can visualize it completely.

What you're really doing is a sort of mental dress rehearsal. By visualizing the entire experience positively, you get comfortable with it, which reduces your stress level and helps you perform well when the actual event happens. The more visualizing you do, the more relaxed you will be.

Remove stressors. OK, I know this sounds simplistic, but one good way to get rid of stress in your life is to get rid of the things that are causing the stress. I don't mean quit your job or divorce your spouse (although those are certainly options). I mean do simple things that can eliminate some stressors. If driving to and from work each day stresses you out, look for alternatives. Maybe you could take public transportation or carpool, or transfer to a job site closer to home.

I have a 50-mile commute in Long Island, New York—one of the most congested areas in the country. Traffic or bad weather can sometimes make this a two-hour journey. However, I have controlled the situation so that it gives me zero stress. First, I chose a thrifty, safe, environmentally friendly *Prius*. Next, I always allow two hours for the one-hour trip. (This way I am always early and never late.) Finally, I use the time to listen to hundreds of books on tape. What a marvelous experience! I have "read" novels, nonfiction, and self-help books during my commute. I have taken a potentially stressful situation, controlled it, and converted the commute into a positive event.

Instead of feeling overwhelmed by everything you have to do, give some thought to what your real priorities are—and then spend your time on those. By managing your time better, you'll be more productive, and you'll have more time for yourself and your family. Most important of all, I think, is learning to say no. Commit yourself only to things that are genuinely important to you. It's all too easy to get sucked into things that will take a lot of your time and energy and leave you feeling stressed instead of satisfied.

Have a drink. Alcohol in moderate amounts is an enjoyable way to both relieve stress and help your heart health. When stress is getting to you, having one drink—and only one—can help. What's a drink? Twelve ounces of beer, three ounces of wine, or one ounce of hard alcohol, such as vodka. That's all. Of course, if you decide to have an alcoholic drink, do so only when you know you can relax—when you have at least two hours in which you don't have to drive anywhere or do anything that requires careful concentration. We know from numerous studies that people who regularly drink alcohol in moderation have a lower risk of heart disease than do people who refrain from drinking entirely.[64] It's probably because the alcohol relaxes your blood vessels, lowers blood pressure, and improves circulation to the heart. Of course, we also know that people who drink heavily have a much greater risk of heart disease (and numerous other health problems). Alcohol is a really good example of how too much of a good thing can be harmful.

Recent studies also suggest that having more than one or two drinks a day can increase a woman's risk of breast cancer.[65] The increase in risk is actually quite small, but there also are other health risks associated with having more than two drinks a day. Why risk it? For most people—male and female—one drink a day is enough to reduce stress and benefit your heart.

There are lots of other stress-reduction techniques you can try. Some people find aromatherapy helpful; others like massages or soaks in a hot tub; for some, meditation or prayer is the answer. Keep trying until you find techniques that work for you, and then make the time to put them into practice on a regular basis.

Finally, remember that people who are under a lot of stress often withdraw from their social lives—and that makes them feel isolated and even more stressed. Social activities are great stress-busters. When you get together with your friends and family, you feel connected, and that can help you get some much-needed perspective on whatever is stressing you.

CHAPTER 5

Exercise Right

Eat right, brush your teeth, wash your hands, reduce your stress level—all those things are crucial to achieving and maintaining good health. But even all of those steps aren't enough. You also need to be physically active.

Why Sweat It?

Exercise is the cornerstone of healthy living. We know from a lot of recent research that your overall fitness level is the single most important predictor of your health and quality of life.[66] And that's true at any age. In general, the fitter you are, the higher your quality of life. And the fitter you are, the longer you are likely to maintain a high level of physical and mental functioning as you get older.

The list of health benefits from regular exercise is actually pretty amazing. Here's what being physically active can do for you:

- Maintain your weight. Exercise helps keep off the creeping weight gains that come with age. If you've lost weight, exercise helps you keep it off. And if you need to lose weight, exercise helps it come off faster.
- Reduce your risk of heart disease. Physical activity raises your beneficial HDL cholesterol and improves your overall blood circulation.

- Lower your blood pressure. Not only does regular exercise reduce your risk of high blood pressure, it can help lower your blood pressure if it's too high.
- Lower your risk of diabetes. Regular physical activity helps maintain your blood sugar at normal levels. If you already have diabetes, exercise improves insulin sensitivity and helps bring down high blood sugar.
- Prevent cancer. If you're the sedentary type, you have an increased risk of colon cancer. Exercise also may help prevent breast cancer. Exercise during cancer treatment helps patients feel better and helps relieve treatment-related fatigue.
- Strengthen your bones. Regular weight-bearing exercise help build and maintain lifelong strong bones.
- Reduce menopause symptoms. Even mild to moderate exercise can reduce the anxiety and depression symptoms that frequently accompany menopause.
- Make you stronger. The increased blood flow and training help muscles become larger and stronger. Strong muscles can help prevent back injuries and protect your joints from arthritis. For older adults, strong muscles mean being able to perform all the usual activities of daily living more easily, and remaining independent longer. And because muscles are more metabolically active than fat, the more muscles you have, the more calories you burn. It's automatic weight control.
- Improve your mental health. Exercise more, and you'll improve your mental health while lowering your risk of anxiety or depression. Exercise also helps you handle stress better, and helps you sleep better.

Have I listed enough reasons? If not, here's the best thing exercise can do for you:

- Improve your longevity. If you exercise briskly and regularly, you could add three years to your life. The highest risk of premature death and disability is found among those who don't engage in regular physical activity.[67]

An article published in the *Archives of Internal Medicine* in 2007 says it all: "People who engage in 20 minutes of vigorous exercise at least three times a week cut their risk of [premature] death by 32 percent." Smaller amounts of exercise still cut risk of death by 19 percent![68]

It's never too late to start an exercise program. Back in 1990, I read a study in the *Journal of the American Medical Association* about a group of elderly nursing home residents who undertook weight training.[69] These men and women were in their 80s and 90s, and all were frail. Yet in just eight weeks, they all showed amazing improvement in muscle strength—up to 157 percent. In fact, some of them no longer needed their walkers! If a bunch of 90-year-olds can become more fit, so can you.

Getting Started

Now that you know all the good reasons for regular exercise, it's time to figure out how much and what kind of exercise you need. Here's the short answer: Walk for 30 minutes at least three times a week. It's easy, you already know how to do it, and it's free.

The long answer will take the rest of this chapter, because 30 minutes three times a week is really just a good starting point. The more you exercise, the more you benefit. For overall good health, and to avoid weight gain, what you really need is 30 to 60 minutes of physical activity on most days of the week. To lose weight, or to keep off weight once you've lost it, your goal should be 60 minutes on most days.

Now that I've said that, let me qualify it a bit. If you're really sedentary, studies show that even 10 minutes of exercise a day will boost your heart health and your overall fitness, especially if you're overweight or obese. Once you can handle 10 minutes a day and you start feeling the benefits, it's not that hard to move on to 11 minutes a day, and to go up from there. The important thing is taking that first step.

Before you begin your exercise program, review the previous chapter, "Think Right." New research suggests that a positive attitude may take some of the aches and pains out of vigorous exercise. According to a study published in the *Journal of Pain,* women who had positive attitudes reported less pain while exercising to their maximum on a stationary bike.[70]

What Kind of Exercise?

For your overall health, your exercise needs to fall into two basic categories: aerobic and strength training.

Aerobic exercise is the kind that gets your heart beating faster, which is why it's also often called cardio exercise. Examples of aerobic exercise include walking briskly, jogging, running, swimming, biking, rollerblading, dancing—anything that raises your heartbeat. You can even meet your exercise goals with housework. Washing windows counts as moderate aerobic activity; so does washing the car or vacuuming the house.

Strength training—also called anaerobic exercise—builds muscles through resistance. Weightlifting, yoga, and tai chi are examples of this type of exercise. By building up your muscles, you increase your overall strength, which makes daily living easier—it's less effort to carry groceries in from the car, for example. Having more muscles also raises your overall metabolic rate, meaning you burn more calories even when you're sitting still. This, in turn, makes it easier to keep your weight under control without counting every calorie. And, of course, strength training also gives you a toned body and makes you feel strong. The best part of strength training: you don't have to do it every day. A 20-minute strength workout twice a week is enough to make your muscles noticeably stronger.

Since aerobic exercise is the kind you should do almost every day, let's get a better idea of what's involved.

For aerobic exercise to be most helpful, it should be moderately intense. That means your heart should beat noticeably faster. You can use a complex formula to figure out exactly how many beats a minute you want to achieve, or you can use the much simpler "talk-sing test." If you can carry on a conversation while exercising, but don't have enough breath to sing, your heart rate is about right. When you walk briskly (about a mile in 15 minutes); do light yard work, such as raking leaves; play tag with your children; or bike at a casual pace, you're getting moderate aerobic exercise.

Vigorous aerobic exercise raises your heart rate more and makes you breathe harder and faster. Examples include jogging or running; swimming laps; rollerblading at a brisk pace; cross-country skiing; or playing a sport like tennis, basketball, soccer, or touch football.

For any fitness activity, you can figure out if you're working hard enough by rating it on a scale of "no effort" to "maximum effort." For aerobic activity, you want to feel that your effort is somewhat hard—whatever that means for you. For some people, a somewhat hard effort might be just walking along slowly on flat ground. For others, somewhat hard might mean walking fast uphill. There's no right answer—it's what feels somewhat hard to *you.*

With strength training, you want to put in more effort. *Gradually* work your way up to feeling that your effort is hard or even very hard. It's the only way to build muscle effectively. To get an idea of what a hard effort is, it helps to know what your maximum level is. You can figure that out by carefully lifting the heaviest weight you can. Then compare how that feels with the way a somewhat lesser effort feels. When it comes to strength training, pushing yourself a little—but carefully, to avoid injury—pays off. Once you start putting in more than a moderate amount of effort, your strength probably will increase rapidly.

As you become more fit, you'll need less effort to accomplish the same amount of exercise. You might decide just to maintain your fitness at that level. That's fine as far as it goes—you'll still be getting plenty of benefit. But why not challenge yourself and become even more fit? It doesn't have to take more time—just more effort. Try walking faster, or change your route to add in some hills. If you're using exercise equipment, such as an exercise bike or a treadmill, increase the resistance. For weight training, gradually add more weight—not more repetitions. Once you're able to lift a weight twelve to fifteen times in a row, add enough weight at the next session so that you can only lift it eight times. Use this weight until it gets too easy, then repeat the addition step.

Fitting in Fitness

I can hear you moaning and groaning. "Thirty minutes a day? Plus two strength-training sessions a week? How am I supposed to fit that into my schedule?" Frankly, of all the excuses for not getting exercise, I find the time factor the least convincing. The average American spends four hours a day watching TV. Surely you can spare at least a half-hour a day away from the tube. If you really can't tear yourself away, then ride an exercise bike, do aerobics, lift weights, or find some other form of activity you can do while watching. Or combine the two: work out with an exercise video!

Your daily 30 minutes don't have to be done all at once. A lot of scientific evidence shows that two 15-minute activity periods, or three 10-minute ones—even if they're hours apart—are just as good as one, solid 30-minute session. That means you can easily get your daily activity by working it into your day, rather than trying to find half an hour in your busy day. I call this "unlazy" exercise. Instead of a scheduled workout, be unlazy and find ways to add some activity throughout your day. Try some of these unlazy ideas:

- Walk up and down the stairs in your house for 10 minutes. Or do it at work during your lunch break.
- Get off the bus or train a stop earlier and walk the rest of the way.
- Leave your car as far away as you can in a parking lot or garage. (Bonus: fewer dings from other drivers.)

- Walk around your block a couple of times.
- Walk once around the shopping mall before you go into any stores.

Remember that your short interval of extra activity has to be continuous for best results. Just taking the stairs instead of an escalator is a beginning, but you need least 10 minutes of exercise to get the greatest benefit.

Getting Strong

Strength or resistance training is the other half of your fitness program. In this type of exercise, your muscles work against some kind of resistance—an applied force or weight. It could be weights, workout bands, or even your own body (pushups are a good example). Strength training builds up both your muscles and your bones. It also helps you improve your balance and coordination, which, in turn, can keep you from having the sort of bad fall that leads to torn ligaments, broken bones, and concussions.

How strong do you need to be? Exercise experts generally suggest a workout routine that includes eight to twelve repetitions of six to eight strength exercises. Twice a week is enough. In fact, strength training is something you don't want to do more than two or three times a week— your muscles need recovery time between workouts.

You don't have to join a gym or buy an expensive machine to get a good strength training workout. Free weights—dumbbells and ankle weights—are inexpensive and easy to use right at home. The same is true for exercise bands and other simple resistance equipment. If possible, however, work with a personal trainer—at least at first, Your trainer can help get you started on a sensible program and teach you how to use your equipment safely and effectively. Check with your local health clubs, YMCAs, and other organizations to find someone. It's money well spent.

NEAT Ideas

Researchers always have wondered why some people seem to stay naturally slimmer and more fit than others, even when they seem to be just as sedentary and eat just as much. Recently researchers at the Mayo Clinic arrived at a good partial explanation: NEAT, or Non-Exercise Activity Thermogenesis. In other words, moving around a lot—or fidgeting.

In the study, participants were outfitted with special clothing that continuously monitored their movements. The researchers found that the calories people burn just through everyday activities are crucial to keeping weight down. Many people are heavy because they naturally tend to move less, so they burn fewer calories—as much as 150 calories a day. It's not the other way around: they don't move less because they're too heavy, although being heavy does worsen the problem by making it harder to move.

If you're not naturally fidgety, you'll have to make a conscious effort to move more. Try these unlazy ideas:

- Park farther away than you usually do.
- Instead of sending email to coworkers, walk down the hall and talk to them instead.
- Always stand when talking on the phone. You burn 30 percent more calories standing rather than sitting. Better yet, use a cordless or cell phone and pace while speaking.
- Take the stairs instead of an escalator or elevator.
- Walk the dog a little farther. Or put your purchases into a hand-basket instead of a shopping cart.

A few years ago, my family was sitting and talking at the table after dinner. My teenage niece had her legs crossed and was nervously shaking her dangling foot. Her mother asked her what she was doing. Without missing a beat, the teenager replied, "I'm burning calories, Mom."

Adding NEAT to your life isn't an alternative to your 30-minute minimum of daily exercise, but it is a good way to get in some additional calorie-burning activity.

A Step in the Right Direction

Going for your daily (I hope) walk is pretty straightforward. The basics are simple: Wear comfortable shoes, dress for the weather, and choose a safe place to walk. Beyond that, there are a few other points to keep in mind:

- Stretch. Before you start and after you're done, do some light stretching exercises.
- Warm up and cool down. Warm up by walking slowly for the first five minutes, then speed up to a brisker pace. Cool down by walking more slowly for the last five minutes.
- Stand up straight and swing your arms naturally as you walk. Standing up helps improve your posture and keep you balanced as you walk. Swinging your arms is part of your body's natural walking motion, and helps to burn more calories.
- Drink water. Have a drink of water before you start out, and carry a water bottle with you. Drink as soon as you start to feel just slightly thirsty.
- Be careful. Let someone know when you're going out for a walk and when you think you'll be back. Carry a cell phone just in case. If you like to wear headphones while you walk, keep the sound low enough so that you can still hear what's going on around you. Whenever possible, choose a low-traffic location, such as a park or shopping mall, for your walk.

Ten Thousand Steps

Your 30 to 60 minutes of daily exercise are in addition to your normal daily activity. You've already read about two ways to fit fitness into your life. You can consciously decide to add exercise to your life in a scheduled way, such as by going for a daily walk or taking an exercise class. Or you can add activity in smaller chunks throughout the day.

There's also a third way: take 10,000 steps a day.

Whoa—10,000 steps! Isn't that an awful lot of walking? Not really. It takes about 2,000 steps to make a mile, so, in theory, 10,000 steps means walking about five miles a day. In reality, you count every step you take all day long toward your daily 10,000. That includes all the steps in your normal daily activities. For the average person, anywhere from 1,000 to 3,000 steps are almost automatic. To get the total higher than that, you need to add in steps. Every single one you take, deliberately or just as part of your usual life, counts toward the total.

It sounds daunting, but it's actually fairly easy to nudge your total daily steps toward 10,000. All those little tricks to increase activity, such as parking farther away or walking short distances instead of driving, add steps. Of course, taking a walk does, too. Exercising in other ways, such as swimming or jogging, count toward the daily total. Estimate them as equivalent to the distance you would walk in the same time. For instance, if you walk a mile in 15 minutes—a moderate pace—that means you take about 2,000 steps in 15 minutes. So, if you jog, swim, or take an aerobics class for half an hour, that would count as 4,000 steps. At that rate you'll be at 10,000 steps in no time!

To track your steps, get an inexpensive pedometer from any sports store. Wear it clipped to your waist, and track your daily steps for a week or two. Averaging the numbers will give you a good idea of your daily activity and how many more steps you need to add. The fun begins when you start tracking your daily steps and thinking up creative new ways to achieve your goal. The bonus comes when you realize that walking 10,000 steps a day helps improve your fitness and keep your weight under control.

At Home or at the Club?

An objection I often hear is that joining a health club is expensive. Who says you have to pay money to exercise? Walking is free (OK, you do have to pay for pair of good shoes), and you don't need walking lessons or a walking coach. Most other forms of exercise also can easily be done at home for nothing. You don't have to spend money on gas, membership fees, or expensive workout clothing, and you get to exercise in the privacy and convenience of your own home.

On the other hand, many people enjoy getting out of the house and being with other people while they exercise. They also find it easier to plan their exercise around a schedule of classes or training sessions at a club—and of course, knowing that you've paid for the membership and the trainer can motivate you to get your money's worth. Working out with a friend or taking an exercise class can be fun. Your exercise buddies can inspire you to try harder and keep you coming back. Health clubs also offer a range of expensive exercise equipment that most people don't have the money or space to have at home. Plus, some clubs offer indoor pools for swimming and water exercise. They also usually offer a range of classes, such as dance aerobics and yoga, that help keep exercise from becoming dull and routine. Some clubs even offer babysitting.

The choice is yours, but remember: it's not an either/or situation. There may be days when getting to the health club is inconvenient or impossible due to a hectic schedule, bad weather, travel, and all the other unexpected things that pop up in life. Having an exercise routine you can do at home keeps you active when the gym just isn't a possibility.

If you do decide to join a health club, there are some important points to consider before you sign the contract:

- Location. Choose a club that's easy to get to from your home or workplace. If you have to go out of your way to get there, you may stop going.
- Facilities. Visit all the local clubs to check out the facilities. The club should be spacious, clean, and well-ventilated. Dirty towels piled in corners in the locker room are not a good sign.
- Equipment. Look for modern, well-maintained exercise equipment. Be sure there's enough of it. You don't want to have to wait to use it or be constrained by time limits during busy periods.

- Hours and class schedule. Most clubs open early and stay open late. Look for a club that offers a good mix of exercise classes at a variety of fitness levels—and at times that are convenient for you.
- Atmosphere. You should feel comfortable at your health club. Look for friendly, supportive, well-trained instructors and a relaxed atmosphere. If you get the feeling that you would have to join another health club in order to get in shape to join the one you're looking at, it's probably not right for you. Many women feel more at ease in women-only health clubs, or at least in one that offers women-only classes and has female instructors.
- Cost. Health-club memberships can be expensive. Before you sign up for a costly year-long membership, ask for a day pass or trial membership to be sure you're happy with your choice. A month-to-month arrangement may be better for you than a year-long commitment. Clubs often offer two-for-one specials. If you and a friend or partner have been talking about joining a gym, these could be good deals. Joining with an exercise buddy can help keep you both motivated. Some clubs throw in all sorts of free stuff, but always read the fine print. Also, check with your boss. Companies sometimes arrange discounts at health clubs for their employees—or your employer may even chip in on some of the cost.

Shop around to find the right health club. Be sure to visit at the times you're most likely to be there. You'll want to know if the club gets crowded or classes fill up too quickly then.

An alternative to a health-club membership is to sign up for yoga, Pilates, tai chi, or some other specific exercise program with a private studio. The financial arrangement is usually less formal than a health club. You can usually pay for a fixed number of classes in advance, or just pay for the classes you take.

Before you sign up with a pricey private health club or exercise studio, check out some low-cost alternatives that can get you out of the house and exercising. Your local recreation center or YMCA/YWCA are possibilities. Another good alternative is a walking group. There are a lot of these. Some are informal—just a group of friends who get together regularly to walk in the neighborhood or at a shopping mall. Others are more organized and are put together by groups such as health clubs, YMCA/YWCAs, churches, or local health providers and hospitals. Ask around in your community, and chances are good you'll find a group to join. If not, start one!

You might decide to spend the money for a gym membership on some home exercise equipment instead. Good choice—but be careful. Don't get caught by a "muscle hustle." When choosing your equipment, be skeptical of the claims the manufacturer makes. Can you really lose several inches from your waist or drop 10 pounds by using the equipment for just a week? No. Can you really get long-lasting results without sweating? No. You don't get the benefits of exercise unless you exercise. Can you burn off fat from a specific part of your body? No again.

Read the fine print carefully before you buy. In addition to being skeptical of claims about effectiveness, check out the payment plan and any "money-back" guarantees carefully. What sounds like a bargain price might not be once you add in the shipping and handling, sales tax, and delivery and set-up fees. Returning the equipment might cost almost as much.

The safest way to buy high-quality exercise equipment isn't to order a gimmick you see on late-night television. Visit a good sports store to see—and try—the equipment for yourself. Also check out the classified ads in local papers for used exercise equipment. A lot of it turns out to be practically brand-new—the heaviest use a lot of home equipment gets is as a place to hang wet towels. You might find a real bargain.

Be on the Safe Side

Every book and article about getting started on an exercise program always advises you to check with your doctor first. Good idea, especially if any of these conditions apply to you:

- You have heart disease or have had a stroke, or are at high risk for them.
- You have diabetes, or are at high risk for it.
- You're obese (BMI over 30—see chapter 3 for more information).
- You have an injury or joint problem, such as arthritis in your knee.
- You're older than age 50.
- You're pregnant.

Even if any of these are true for you, your doctor will almost certainly still encourage you to exercise—just with some cautions. If you have knee arthritis, for instance, water aerobics might be better for you than walking because it puts less stress on your joints. Even people who have serious disabilities can improve their heart health, lung capacity, strength, mobility, flexibility, and coordination by staying physically active. If you have heart disease, your doctor might actually prescribe exercise—and your health insurance might even pay for it. Recent studies have shown that exercise is extremely helpful for people with congestive heart failure.

To avoid injury while exercising, use your common sense. Start any new exercise program gradually, especially if you haven't exercised on a regular basis much until now. Always begin your workout with a warm-up or some stretching; end with a cool-down period or more stretching. Wear comfortable clothes and appropriate footwear. When using exercise equipment, make sure it's working properly and is adjusted correctly for your height and ability level. If you have chest pain or feel breathless, dizzy, nauseous, or faint while exercising, stop and rest—and call for medical help, if necessary.

If you take walks, follow basic precautions. Don't walk in traffic or in bad neighborhoods, wear reflective clothing if you walk at night, and carry a cell phone in case of problems.

It's important not to wimp out on your exercise program. But it's also important to know the difference between the mild muscle soreness and stiffness you might feel the next day—what personal trainers often call "good pain"—and a real injury. Ditto for the discomfort you might feel in an arthritic joint. As a general rule, if a muscle or joint really hurts; hurts a lot more than usual; or is swollen, red, or warm to the touch, you've been overdoing it. For self-care, follow the RICE rule: Rest, ice, compress (with an elastic bandage), and elevate. If you have severe pain or significant swelling, or if the pain doesn't start to get better within 24 hours, you may have an injury that needs medical attention. Don't delay.

Staying Motivated

Time after time, I see people start out on a good exercise program and gradually abandon it, even when the exercise has helped them lose weight and feel better. This always puzzles me, because regular exercise makes me feel so much better that I can't imagine not doing it. In fact, when I miss more than day, I really notice the difference in my physical sense of well-being and also in my mood and energy level. I think many people who give up on their fitness programs haven't really incorporated exercise into their lives. They see it as a daily chore instead of something pleasurable, or as something that they will do just until they "get into shape."

Make your exercise enjoyable and interesting. That's the best way you can help yourself stay motivated to do it. Like a lot of other people, I like to watch the news while exercising at home on my elliptical trainer or rowing machine. A friend of mine prefers to listen to recorded books. He says that helps him exercise his brain along with his body. He's certainly well-read (or maybe that should be well-listened). Exercising with a family member or friend can make the time pass pleasantly. You may even enjoy being with them so much that you add some extra time to your routine—I know I do. And don't forget that your dog can be a great exercise buddy. A fascinating 2008 article in the *American Journal of Public Health* showed that physical activity and walking were 57 to 77 percent higher in dog owners compared to non-dog owners![71]

Exercise for Children

I see a lot of children and teenagers in my orthodontic practice. Some of them are real jocks—they play on all sorts of organized teams. Most aren't. In fact, most of them don't play any sports at all, unless video games count. When I ask them about phys ed class, they tell me that they only have it once or twice a week—and a surprising number of them manage to get out of it with medical excuses. In a lot of cases, children who are actually interested in playing sports get pressured to give them up to concentrate on their schoolwork.

Every day I speak with children who tell me they are tired, they don't sleep enough, and the only exercise they get is moving their mouse! These children are being set up for a lifetime of inactivity, with all the bad health consequences that go with it. Some of them are already confirmed couch potatoes at the age of 10.

It's absolutely crucial to get our kids off the couch and into physical activity. My slogan is, "No child left indoors."

Physical activity is important for children for almost exactly the same reasons it is for adults. In addition to all the physical reasons—healthy weight, strong muscles, less risk of chronic disease—regular exercise helps children sleep better and have a better outlook on life. They're less anxious and less likely to be depressed.

How much exercise do children need? The current rule of thumb among pediatricians is that for toddlers through to preschoolers, 60 minutes of planned activity plus 60 minutes of free play is about right. School-aged children need an hour or more every day. Once children start school, that hour can be broken up into smaller segments of at least 15 minutes each.

Step one in getting your children to be active is to set a good example by being active yourself. That doesn't mean just doing it; it means being positive about it. If you complain about exercising and make it sound like a chore or punishment, your children aren't going to have a positive approach to exercising, either.

The same children who tell me they don't have time for sports or exercise because they're so busy are the same children who spend hours every day on their computers, playing video games, watching TV, and talking or sending text messages to their friends. (It's possible that I'm also describing you.) Some of that time could be spent being active instead. Limit the time your children—and you—spend in front of electronic screens of various sorts every day. One exception to that rule might be video games that get you moving, such as *Dance Dance Revolution* and *Wii* games. Most experts recommend that children get only one to two hours of screen time—meaning TV, computer, and video games *combined*—per day.

Just as adults can easily add activity to their daily lives, children can, too. Instead of driving the children to the library or to school, or sending them on a bus, let them walk or ride their bikes. Yes, it might take a little more organization, especially at first, but the benefits are worth it. Today school systems are so concerned about sedentary children that they're starting to encourage biking and walking to school. Some schools are now organizing "walking school buses." Groups of children meet at a "walk stop" and are escorted by volunteer parents to the school. Encourage your children to participate in after-school sports programs. Above all, encourage them to just get outside and *play*—whether it's jumping rope, playing tag or catch, bike riding, skating, or any other unstructured activity that's fun and gets them moving. Other fun activities, such as bowling, miniature golf, or going to a batting cage or skate park, are great, too.

What I really enjoy is exercising with my family. We just don't call it that—we call it quality time instead. We go on a family bike ride or for a swim at the beach. It's fun, we get some exercise, and we get to spend some time together without distractions.

No Excuses

Between my patients, my friends, and my family, I've probably heard every excuse there is for not exercising. For every excuse, there's an answer.

- "I'm too busy." OK, maybe there are some days when you really can't squeeze in any exercise. But on most days you can find time—even if it's in 10-minute increments—to work in some exercise.
- "I'm too tired." At the end of a long day, you might well be too tired to work out. But who says you have to wait until the end of the day? Like many other people, I find that exercising in the morning before I go off to work gets me energized for the day. Other people prefer to rev themselves up by exercising at lunch time. And again, if you're too tired for a half-hour workout, try doing just 10 minutes instead. Whenever I do this, I always end up doing the full half hour instead—once I get going, it's hard to stop.
- "I don't need to lose weight, so why bother?" The health benefits of exercise go way beyond weight control. Plus, exercise lifts your mood and increases your energy level. And research shows that people who are overweight, active, and fit actually live longer than people who are of ideal weight but are inactive and unfit.[72]
- "It's boring!" Riding an exercise bike all by yourself down in the basement *is* boring, but it doesn't have to be. Listen to music or an audio book; watch TV; or better yet, ride a real bike outside,

preferably with a friend. Exercise buddies can make the time go much faster.

- "I'm afraid of injuries." It's hard to hurt yourself walking 30 minutes a day at whatever pace is comfortable for you. In general, moderate intensity physical activity is low risk. Try water workouts in a pool if you have joint problems. A personal trainer can help you work out a good exercise program if you have chronic health problems that limit your mobility.
- "I'm not into playing sports." Take walks or use exercise equipment.
- "I can't afford a gym." Fitness is free. Take a walk, work in your garden, clean the house, take the children to the park.
- "It's too hot/too cold/too wet." If you've joined a health club, that excuse is totally out the window. If you haven't, join one or exercise indoors at home. Walking around a shopping mall can be done in any weather.
- "My family and friends aren't supportive." You're exercising for yourself, not for them.

Getting fit is simple. All it takes to get started is literally putting one foot in front of the other. A simple walk of just a few minutes can start you down the path of better health.

One last thought that might help to stimulate you to exercise: a drink a day plus exercise may help you to live longer. In the previous chapter we discussed how one drink a day was useful for reducing stress. New research, published in 2008 in the *European Heart Journal,* shows that while mild drinking is healthy and exercising is healthy, doing a little of both is even healthier![73] Researchers studied the drinking and exercising habits of 12,000 men for a 20-year period. The men who had the lowest risk of dying at young age from any cause were physically active and mild drinkers! And, surprise of all surprises, the highest risk went to those who were physically inactive and heavy drinkers.

CHAPTER 6

Sleep Right

We spend about a third of our lives in bed, but not too many of us today are getting enough sleep. In fact, we're getting less and less sleep—even as we're getting fatter and fatter; developing Type II diabetes, high blood pressure, heart disease, and cancer; and crashing more cars. Is there a connection? Absolutely. We know from a large and growing body of research that getting enough sleep—starting in infancy—is crucial to good health.

Sleep Statistics

A hundred years ago, the average American got nine hours of sleep every night. Today, the average American is sleeping less than seven hours a night. Surveys by the National Institutes of Health and the National Sleep Foundation show that about a third of all adults get so sleepy during the day that it interferes with their ability to work effectively and have a social life. This is what physicians call "problem sleepiness."

A 2007 survey by the National Sleep Foundation found that 60 percent of American women said they only get a good night's sleep a few times a week; 43 percent said daytime sleepiness interferes with their daily activities. On top of that, the Institute of Medicine (IOM) says that anywhere from 50 to 70 million Americans have chronic sleep disorders that keep them from being well rested, hinder their daily functioning, and affect their long-term health.[74]

A little-known aspect of too little sleep is drowsy driving—a problem that may be more prevalent than drunk driving, and is just as dangerous. In fact, the IOM says about 20 percent of all serious car crash injuries are associated with sleepy drivers who didn't drink any alcohol.

Even young children today aren't getting enough sleep. Experts recommend that infants aged 3 to 11 months should sleep 14 to 15 hours a day, but a survey by the National Sleep Foundation discovered that, on average, these babies were sleeping just 13 hours a day. Toddlers should be getting 12 to 14 hours' sleep, but the survey found they were getting just under 12 hours a day. For preschoolers, the recommended amount is 11 to 13 hours; these children average only a bit over 10 hours a day. For schoolchildren up to age 10 or so, the experts suggest 10 to 11 hours of sleep, but the average is just 9.5 hours a night.

As any parent knows, when children don't sleep enough, they show it. Some just get sleepy during the day, but others can become hyperactive, irritable, aggressive, and show other behavior problems. Of course, so can their parents when they don't get enough sleep!

The solution is simple: sleep more, feel better.

Putting that into action is more difficult.

What Is Sleep?

To understand why you need more sleep, or how to get more restful sleep, you need to understand what sleep really is. When you go to sleep, you're not just turning yourself off for a few hours. Your body may be relaxed while you're asleep, but your brain stays active. During any sleep period, you cycle through a distinct series of stages—and each stage is important for sleeping well and feeling well rested when you awake.

Sleep researchers divide sleep into two basic categories: rapid eye movement (REM) sleep, and non-REM sleep (also called slow-wave sleep). During REM sleep, you dream. Your brain is active, and your eyes move rapidly even though they're closed. Your breathing is more rapid, and it's also irregular and shallow. Your heart rate and blood pressure go up. Your arm and leg muscles become temporarily paralyzed, which keeps you from acting out your dreams.

A complete sleep cycle of REM and non-REM sleep generally takes about 90 to 100 minutes, and starts with non-REM sleep. Most people will have between four and five sleep cycles a night.

Non-REM sleep is divided into four stages:

- Stage 1: You're in a light sleep and can be easily awakened. This is the transition state between sleeping and waking. Your muscle activity and eye movements slow down. This stage is short, usually lasting just a few minutes.
- Stage 2: Your eye movements stop; you have slower brain waves with occasional bursts of rapid brain waves; and your body temperature drops a bit. This stage also usually lasts only a few minutes.
- Stage 3: You're in a deep sleep. Waking you at this point would be difficult. Your brain waves are even slower, but you still have some rapid waves.
- Stage 4: The deepest sleep of all. You're very hard to wake. Your brain waves are extremely slow.

During Stages 3 and 4, your breathing slows, and your blood pressure drops. Your body also releases hormones, such as growth hormone, that are important for regulating and repairing your body. Stage 3 and Stage 4 deep sleep are the restorative stages—the ones you need to feel well-rested when you get up in the morning. Overall, you spend about 75 percent of your sleep time in non-REM sleep.

Your first cycle of REM sleep usually happens about 90 minutes after you fall asleep. You do dream during non-REM sleep stages, but the most vivid dreams happen during REM sleep. As the night goes on, you spend less time in Stage 3 and Stage 4 sleep and more time in REM sleep, so you dream for longer periods of time.

What's the purpose of all that dreaming? That's a question that people have been asking for thousands of years, and we still don't know for sure. Even if sleep researchers don't fully understand why you need to dream, they do know it's important. Dreams probably have a lot to do with laying down the brain pathways that are essential for learning and remembering. Research has shown that we learn better if we're well rested, and we remember something better if we study it and then "sleep on it." We also perform better if we're well rested. That sluggish feeling you get if you haven't slept enough—which also means you haven't dreamed enough—affects how you think. Not only does lack of sleep slow down your thinking processes, it also makes it hard to pay attention and stay focused. You get confused easily and are more likely to make bad decisions or take dangerous risks. If you're chronically short of sleep, you're also more likely to be irritable or even downright depressed.

When I was earning my doctorate at Columbia, I spent many evenings at the 24-hour study room at the Columbia Health Science Center Library. Here medical, dental, nursing, and PhD students often studied through the night.

It was here that I discovered the "Trash Can Phenomenon." Students used this room all day and all night. During the day—when the room was actually the busiest—the trash can area was the cleanest. Students tossed their trash into the garbage pails, and if their aim was off, they would get up, pick the trash off the floor, and deposit it where it belonged.

It was a totally different story past midnight. The floors around the cans became dirtier and dirtier. Not because the trash cans were overfilled, but because the students' aim became progressively worse as the evening wore on. And when the exhausted students missed the can, their poor judgment led them to believe that it was OK to just leave the trash there.

Getting in Sync with Sleep

To get a good night's sleep and wake up feeling rested and ready for the day, you need to get in sync with your sleep cycle. We all have a natural sleep and wake cycle. It's regulated by both your internal body clock and external signals. Your biological internal clock is controlled by a complex feedback loop involving brain cells that respond to light signals received through your eyes. When the environment gets darker as night falls, your biological clock triggers the release of the hormone melatonin, which makes you feel sleepy. As the evening and night go on, you release more and more melatonin, which makes you sleepier and sleepier, especially during the early morning hours. As dawn approaches, you stop making melatonin and your body prepares to wake up.

Generally speaking, people feel sleepiest between midnight and seven in the morning; they're at their drowsiest in the early morning hours. (The sleepiness many people feel in the mid-afternoon, often between 1:00 and 4:00 PM, is probably related, at least in part, to a small increase in melatonin production.) That's why shift work and night jobs are so hard on your body—you're fighting your natural tendency to sleep during the hours of darkness. When you try to sleep during the daylight hours, even when you're tired from working, your body still fights back. It's not getting the internal hormonal cues and the external signals it needs to make you feel sleepy and stay asleep through the normal sleep cycles.

How much sleep do you really need? That varies a lot from person to person, and it also varies throughout an individual's lifetime. On average, most adults need the proverbial eight hours, but there are many people who do just fine on seven hours or even less, and there are others who can't get by on less than nine hours or even more. The same is true for people who are early birds and night owls—these patterns seem to be pretty much genetically determined.

I have always been an earlier riser. During my college years, I invariably chose courses that began at 8:00 AM. I had no problem rising at 6:30 or 7:00 AM, going to the dining hall and having a full breakfast, and then going to class feeling fully awake. I enjoyed my days, and would usually go to bed between 11:00 and 11:30 PM

My dormitory neighbor had a different internal body clock than I had. He never chose a class before 11:00 AM and would stay up until early hours of the morning. Once or twice a week, Adam would practice his guitar at about midnight. After 10 or 15 minutes, I would bang on the paper-thin walls and ask him to stop. This scenario continued week after week. Then I had a brilliant idea. Before I went to bed, I rearranged my stereo system. I placed the loudspeakers directly up against the paper-thin wall. The next morning, at exactly 6:30 AM, I played John Philip Sousa's "Stars and Stripes Forever" at full blast. While I don't think I permanently reset Adam's internal body clock, I certainly aquatinted him with *my* body-clock settings. We never spoke about this incident, but his guitar practice was always held at a more reasonable hour after that.

Your sleep pattern changes as you age. Babies and young children spend about half their sleep time in REM sleep. As we age, we dream less. Adults generally spend about 20 to 25 percent of their sleep time in REM sleep. Adults also sleep less deeply. As a general rule, we spend less and less time in Stage 3 and Stage 4 sleep as we get older, and more time in the lighter Stage 1 and Stage 2 sleep. By the time you're 30, the amount of deep sleep you get in a night is about half what you got when you were 20. As you age, you lose even more deep sleep. You also tend to wake up more during the night, and to have more trouble getting back to sleep when you do. By the time you're 65, you spend less than five percent of your sleep time in deep sleep—as compared to about 20 percent when you're 20. Many adults older than age 75 never really get into Stage 4 sleep at all. At the same time, you naturally produce a lot less melatonin, so you may feel less sleepy in the evening and have trouble falling asleep. It's not true, however, that older people need less sleep than they did when they were younger. In fact, because their sleep isn't as restful, they may need to sleep longer at night or take a nap during the day.

Trying to fight your natural sleep length is pretty much a losing battle. If you cut your sleep short, you'll spend less time in bed at night, but you'll end up having a problem with daytime sleepiness instead. On the other hand, sleeping longer won't help if the quality of your sleep is poor. If you're awakened often during the night, your natural REM/non-REM cycle gets disrupted. When that happens, you won't wake up feeling rested even if you've been in bed for longer than eight hours.

Most people have a pretty good idea of how much sleep they need. The problem is that they don't get that amount.

Paying Off Your Sleep Debt

No matter how hard you push yourself and how long you postpone going to bed, at some point you need to sleep. What makes you sleepy is, among other things, a build-up of a natural chemical called adenosine in your bloodstream. When you sleep for long enough, the adenosine is broken down again, and you wake up feeling rested. If you don't sleep long enough, you don't break down all the adenosine, and you wake up still feeling tired or groggy. Keep up the undersleeping for a few days, and you build up a "sleep debt."

Your body wants to react to a sleep debt by making you sleep longer or more deeply the next night. If your sleep debt is small—you had a short night because you were up with a sick child, for instance—you can easily make it up the next night. That's part of your body's natural ability to adapt to those occasional times when you can't get a full night's sleep. But if you run up a big sleep debt, it's not so easy to pay it off. After several nights of undersleeping, you can start to lose the ability to compensate well for the lost hours, even if you sleep late on the weekend or take naps during the day.

Sleeping in on Saturday also won't erase any goofs you made during the week because you were too tired to function well. And if you're chronically short of sleep, the negative impact on your health is very powerful.

Sleep Well to Feel Well

When you frequently stint on sleep, the damage goes a lot deeper than just feeling tired. More and more research shows that lack of sleep is directly related to a long list of serious health problems.

Heart disease. When you sleep, your heart gets a rest and your blood pressure goes down—and the deeper the sleep, the greater the drop. On average, your heart rate and blood pressure decrease by about 10 percent over the course of a night's sleep. That may not sound like much, but it seems to be crucial for heart health. Studies show that without that nightly drop, your risks of stroke, irregular heartbeat, and heart attack go up. So does your risk of congestive heart failure.

It doesn't take much lost sleep to stress your heart. In a 2007 study at the University of Pennsylvania School of Medicine, participants endured just five nights of four hours of sleep a night. The lack of sleep significantly raised their heart rates, putting them at greater risk of high blood pressure and heart disease.[75] In addition, some studies have shown that people who chronically don't get enough sleep have higher blood levels of C-reactive protein (CRP).[76] Although CRP is a somewhat controversial marker of possible heart disease, it is associated with blood vessel inflammation and a greater risk of atherosclerosis, or hardening of the arteries.

What about the recent studies that claim people who sleep more than eight hours actually have a higher risk of premature death? And that those who sleep only seven hours have the lowest risk of death? The studies have to be taken seriously, because they're good ones. They're based on data from three long-running studies, including the famous Nurses' Health Study from Harvard, that have been tracking large groups of people over many years.

What the studies mostly show, however, is that people who naturally sleep between seven and eight hours, instead of eight hours or more, are perfectly normal—they aren't at increased risk of early death or health problems, and they shouldn't try to make themselves sleep longer or take naps. In other words, if you feel most refreshed after sleeping for eight hours, don't set your alarm clock an hour earlier. Likewise, if you feel fine and can get through the day comfortably on a bit less than seven hours of sleep, don't worry. In all the studies, the people who regularly slept less than what was optimum for them—no matter what that number was—were at greater risk of poor health and premature death. In the Nurses' Health Study, for instance, women who regularly slept five or fewer hours had an amazing 83 percent greater chance of developing heart disease than did women who slept between seven and eight hours.

People who sleep longer than eight hours a night may be at greater risk of illness and untimely death because they're actually not sleeping well, even though they're sleeping longer—in fact, they're sleeping longer to try to make up for not sleeping well. And that brings us right back to all the lack-of-sleep factors that increase the risk of heart disease. Again, looking at data from the Nurses' Health Study, the women who regularly slept nine or more hours had a 57 percent greater chance of developing heart disease than did women who slept seven to eight hours.

Just to confuse the issue even more, a 2004 study looked at long sleepers (people who sleep more than eight hours) and short sleepers (those who sleep less than seven hours). Both groups reported sleep problems such as insomnia, frequent waking during the night, and drowsiness during the day.

Obesity. I always used to laugh when I would read those ridiculous ads for weight loss that said things like, "Sleep yourself thin!" or "Lose weight painlessly while you sleep!" It turns out that's not such a ridiculous idea after all.

Chronic lack of sleep may be a big factor in our current epidemic of obesity. Sleep has a powerful effect on the hormones that help control appetite. When you sleep, your body increases its production of the appetite-suppressing hormone leptin, and decreases its production of the appetite-stimulating hormone ghrelin. Sleep less than you should, and your appetite hormones get out of whack. Not only do you feel hungrier when you don't get enough sleep, you also crave high-calorie, high-carbohydrate foods like cookies and French fries. On top of that, because you're so tired, your ability to make good decisions is diminished—so you choose the ice cream instead of the apple.

In study after study, people who only get five or six hours of sleep each night are much more likely to become obese compared to people who regularly sleep seven to eight hours. How much more likely? Well, scientists recently looked at results from the ongoing National Health and Nutrition Examination Survey begun in the 1980s. The follow-up information from the 18,000 participants showed that those who regularly slept less than four hours were 73 percent more likely to be obese than were those who slept seven to eight hours. Those who averaged only five hours' sleep had a 50 percent greater risk of obesity; those who averaged six hours, a 23 percent greater risk.[77]

Type II diabetes. As with obesity, so with Type II diabetes—which is, after all, closely linked to overweight and lack of exercise. And as with obesity, it turns out that lack of sleep also plays a role in Type II diabetes. When you sleep, your blood-sugar levels naturally rise and fall. But if you get too little sleep, the fall part doesn't happen. Looking again at the Nurses' Health Study, we see that the women who slept the least had a greater risk of developing diabetes than other women, even after the figures were adjusted to account for being overweight or obese.[78] Those who slept five or fewer hours a night had an 18 percent greater chance of becoming diabetic than those who slept seven to eight hours. Similar results were found in a 2005 sleep-health study of nearly 1,500 men and women.[79] Those who slept fewer than five hours a night were 2.5 times as likely to develop diabetes as those who slept seven to eight hours. Given the way undersleeping increases your appetite and disrupts your normal blood-sugar changes, the diabetes figure isn't all that surprising.

What's more surprising is that sleeping too much also can lead to diabetes. The women in the Nurses' Health Study who slept nine hours or more a night had a 29 percent greater chance of developing diabetes.

The 2005 sleep-health study reported similar results: participants who slept more than 9 hour per night were 1.7 times as likely to develop diabetes. Researchers are still puzzled by these results. One possible explanation is that many overweight or obese people suffer from sleep apnea (I'll talk more about that later in this chapter). This condition disrupts the sleep pattern and also is known to be related to difficulties in metabolizing blood sugar—which, in turn, can lead to diabetes. These people may sleep longer because they're trying to make up for the disturbed, low-quality sleep caused by the apnea, or because of some other underlying problem that prevents them from getting restorative sleep.

Cancer. The evidence linking lack of sleep and cancer isn't as powerful as it is for heart disease and diabetes, but it still suggests a link. We know that women who work nights have a moderately greater risk of breast cancer. We still don't know exactly why, but one theory is that night work disrupts your production of melatonin. In women, melatonin suppresses estrogen, the female hormone. When estrogen doesn't get suppressed every night, you end up with too much of it—and high estrogen levels are associated with a greater risk of breast cancer. Not sleeping enough would have the same disruptive effect on melatonin.

Crash in Bed, Not on the Road

Clever slogan, right? I can't claim credit for it—it comes from the people who study sleep and accidents at the National Institutes of Health.[80] The slogan neatly sums up a serious problem: drowsy driving.

It's hard to say exactly how many car crashes involve drivers who can't stay alert behind the wheel. Unlike alcohol-related crashes, there's no breathalyzer test for drowsiness, and many states don't track drowsy-driver accidents the way they do drunk-driving ones. Even so, the U.S. National Highway Traffic Safety Administration estimates conservatively that at least 71,000 people are injured in drowsy-driving accidents every year.[81] And that's just the people who are hurt when a driver actually falls asleep at the wheel. It doesn't begin to estimate the number injured because a driver is awake, but too tired to react quickly. We know that when sleep-deprived people are tested in a driving simulator, they perform as badly—or worse—as they would if they were drunk. Combine lack of sleep with alcohol, and you get a very dangerous driver.

For more on drowsy driving and steps to take to prevent it, please see Chapter 7.

Sleepy Teens

Teenagers need plenty of sleep—nine hours a night is recommended—but they're not getting it. It's not just that teens today often have heavy schoolwork loads plus part-time jobs that eat into their time. The underlying problem is that the hormonal shifts of puberty—especially the increased production of both melatonin and sex hormones—make teenagers sleepy later in the evening than both younger children and most adults. They also want to sleep later in the morning, as anyone who has tried to get a teenager up for school knows. Because school systems completely ignore the reality of teens' sleep patterns, most high schools start early. Having to get up early for school when they went to bed late cuts the average sleep time of a teenager today to about seven hours a night.

I treat thousands of teenagers each year in my orthodontic office. It amazes me how many of them tell me that they're tired. Whether it's eight in the morning or eight in the evening, when I ask a teen, "How are you doing?" quite frequently the response is, "I'm tired!"

"A young, healthy kid like you? Why are you so tired?" I ask. Then I hear the reasons. Up all night playing computer games. Text messaging friends at 2:00 AM. Sleepovers. *Simpsons* reruns.

It really was easier to get enough sleep when I was a kid—there were far fewer distractions. After 11:00 PM, there was nothing to do. No cell phones, no computers, no cable TV. The only thing on network TV was the news, and what teenager wants to watch that? The only choice was reading or sleeping. Most of us chose sleep!

Not sleeping enough has the same effects on teens as it does on adults. Among other things, teens who don't sleep enough are more likely to be overweight or obese.

Of great concern is a 2004 report in the respected medical journal *Sleep*. According to the study, teens who routinely didn't get enough sleep were at higher risk for suicidal thoughts and attempted suicide.[82] Other studies have shown that children and teens with depressive disorders also often have sleep disorders.

I know from my own two teenagers that it's almost impossible to get them to slow down and sleep more. Between school, after-school sports and other activities, part-time jobs, computer time, and hanging with their friends, children have a lot to keep up with. Sleep tends to be low on the priority list. But when teens don't get enough sleep, one of the first things to suffer is their schoolwork. They can start to have real problems with concentration and mood.

To get your teens to sleep longer and better, you must remove all distractions. The rule has got to be this: after 11:00 PM, no computers, no TV, no iPods, no electronics. Read or sleep. That's the choice. Use your parental powers to enforce this rule, and stick to it! And try applying it to yourself as well—you may be amazed at how much better you feel, too.

How to Get a Good Night's Sleep

Getting a good night's sleep is simple. It's a matter of good sleep hygiene—or, in simpler terms, common sense. For now, let's assume that you're an ordinary person trying to get seven or eight hours of restful sleep on an ordinary night. (There are certainly plenty of exceptions to the ordinary, so I'll discuss sleep problems later in this chapter.)

Here are my top ten tips for sleeping well:

1. *Set up a sleep schedule and stick to it.* That means going to bed and getting up at the same time every day, weekends and days off included. Your body really prefers to have a regular sleep

pattern. If you know that you'll be heading to bed at pretty much the same time every night, you can apply the other ideas for getting good sleep more successfully, because most of them depend on a regular schedule.

2. *No caffeine for at least four hours before bedtime!* You'd think this would be pretty obvious—and it is, for beverages like coffee and tea. What many people don't realize, however, is that caffeine is in a lot of other drinks, especially colas and some herbal teas. It's also added to some soft drinks, like Mountain Dew (caffeine is the only drug that can legally be added to food). There's also some natural caffeine in chocolate. Most people clear caffeine from their system in about four to six hours, though it can linger in some people for up to eight hours. So, if you have a late-afternoon cup of coffee at 4:00 pm, it could still keep you up at bedtime. A cup of coffee after dinner is even more likely to do so.

3. *No alcohol for at least four hours before bedtime!* OK, a nightcap can help you relax and fall asleep, but that's deceptive. Alcohol disrupts your sleep pattern and interferes with both deep sleep and REM sleep. When you drink alcohol before sleeping, you never get into the most restful sleep stages. In addition, when the effect of the alcohol wears off a few hours later, you'll probably wake up and have a hard time getting back to sleep.

4. *No big meals before bed.* A light snack, especially if it contains both some protein and complex carbohydrates (say, peanut butter on whole-wheat crackers) will satisfy your hunger and help you sleep. A big meal, however, can cause indigestion or heartburn that will interfere with sleep.

5. *No late-night beverages.* Drinking a lot of liquids before sleep can make you awaken to urinate. If you find that a warm bedtime drink helps you relax, go ahead, but try to limit the total amount of fluids you take in during the late evening.

6. *No smoking.* You might think that's the ultimate no-brainer for

a lot of reasons, not the least of which being the danger of fire from smoking in bed. But you may not realize that nicotine also is a stimulant that can seriously disrupt your sleep pattern. Smokers don't sleep deeply.

7. *Get plenty of exercise.* But don't exercise within two or three hours—or more, for some people—of bedtime. Exercise is stimulating, which is good, but you may not settle down in time to relax for sleep.

8. *Relax before bedtime.* That's probably the easiest thing to say and one of the hardest to do, because we're all so overscheduled and have so many easy distractions nearby. Even so, good sleep depends a lot on unwinding as bedtime approaches. Stop working, get off the phone, and turn off the TV or computer at least half an hour before you plan to sleep. Read a book, listen to music, or do something else that relaxes you.

9. *Take a hot bath before bedtime.* Yes, it's a form of relaxation, but there's more to it than that. After a bath your body temperature drops a bit, which helps you feel sleepy.

10. *Set up your bedroom for good sleep.* Ideally, your bedroom should be quiet, dark, and cool, with a comfortable mattress and pillow. Anything that keeps you up or distracts you from your regular bedtime is out—and that usually means the TV and computer.

Stop the Snoring

While we're on top ten lists, let's talk about the number-one sleep myth: snoring is normal. Occasional snoring is common, especially as we get older, but frequent, loud snoring isn't normal at all.

When you sleep, your soft palate (the soft tissue behind the roof of your mouth), your tongue, and your throat all relax. This narrows or partially blocks the airways at the back of your mouth and in your upper throat. The increased air turbulence makes the soft tissues in your throat vibrate. In other words, you snore. Most people snore every now and then, but if you have allergies or sinus problems, or if you're over-weight, you're more likely to snore. Alcohol and sedatives taken before sleep also relax those areas and can make you snore more.

Snoring might be the subject of a lot of jokes, but it's a serious mat-ter. When you snore, you have to work harder to get enough air, which can disrupt your sleep pattern and lead to problem sleepiness during the day. Snoring also is associated with an increased risk of diabetes, even if you're not overweight. And, it also may raise your risk of high blood pressure, stroke, and heart failure. Snoring in children has been linked to hyperactivity and lower intelligence.[83]

In some people, snoring is a lot more than just an annoyance to their bed partner: it's sleep apnea. This condition results when the soft tissue at the back of the throat partially or completely blocks the air-way. When that happens, you stop breathing briefly, usually for about 10 to 20 seconds. The blockage usually happens *20 to 30 times or more every hour* that you're asleep. Each time, the blockage keeps you from getting enough oxygen. Your brain then responds to the low oxygen by waking you up just enough to open up the airway, but not enough to make you waken fully. You start to breathe normally, often with loud snort or a choking sound, and you go back to sleep—at which point the whole process starts all over again. The upshot is that you never spend enough time in the deep sleep stages, so you never wake up feeling well rested and you often have trouble with excessive sleepiness during the day.

Some 12 to 18 million American adults have sleep apnea. It's more common in men than in women, and more than half of all people who have sleep apnea are overweight.[84] A lot of children have sleep apnea too, often because they have enlarged tonsils and adenoids. These chil-dren are at risk of being misdiagnosed as hyperactive or having atten-tion-deficit disorder, when all they really need is better sleep.

When you have sleep apnea, the disruption to your sleep cycle has the same bad effects as any other kind of disruption, including increases in blood pressure and blood sugar. About a third of all people who have Type II diabetes also have sleep apnea. It's possible that for some, their problems with blood sugar and blood pressure are due to the apnea. In any case, fixing the apnea problem can help get blood sugar and blood pressure problems under control.

Treatment of the occasional snoring problem largely consists of having someone nudge you in the night and say, "Roll over, dear." You snore most when you sleep on your back, so often just turning onto your side turns off the noise.

Chronic snorers can sometimes benefit from dental devices that reposition the jaw and tongue. These types of appliances, which can be constructed by your dentist, hold the lower jaw forward and slightly open, thus improving the air flow through the trachea. Snoring is sometimes completely eliminated.

This has saved at least one marriage that I know of. The husband's snoring was so bad that he had to sleep in a separate room from his wife. He refused surgery, and the snoring and associated sleep deprivation were causing heightened anxiety and tension. It was ruining their marriage. An inexpensive anti-snoring appliance did the trick! His snoring was almost entirely eliminated, and they are back in the same room.

There are a lot of other snoring "remedies" out there, such as nasal strips and special mouth and throat sprays, but there's not a lot of evidence that they work. If you're overweight, slimming down will probably help quite a bit. So will avoiding alcohol and other sedatives at night, and giving up smoking. Clearing up chronic congestion from allergies also may be helpful. Children who snore because of swollen tonsils and adenoids may need surgery to correct the problem.

Sleep apnea treatment is a little more involved. First, you need to be diagnosed with the problem, which is usually done by spending a night being monitored at a sleep lab. If sleep apnea is identified, the usual treatment is a "continuous positive airway pressure" (CPAP) device.

This is a mask that fits over your nose or mouth and continuously blows a gentle stream of air into your airway to keep it open while you sleep. It takes a little getting used to, but CPAP is a very effective treatment. If you suspect you have sleep apnea, talk to your doctor.

Napping

There used to be a lot of not-so-restful arguing among sleep specialists about the value of napping. Most agreed that the occasional nap is helpful, especially if your sleep was interrupted the night before, but there was a lot of disagreement about the value of regular napping. Some even argued that it was bad for your health.

More and more, however, sleep experts are coming down on the plus side of napping as a way to re-energize during the day, even if you slept well the night before. Most people have a natural dip in energy in the mid-afternoon that correlates to a natural dip in melatonin production. That's one reason the siesta is such an established pattern in many countries. Fighting the urge to nap may actually be counterproductive. You still feel the desire to sleep, and that sleepiness can lead to irritability, mistakes at work, bad judgments, and other problems.

Recent research also suggests that men who nap regularly have a markedly lower risk of heart disease.[85] This finding comes from a major long-term European study of nutrition and cancer, so it's a little surprising—the researchers weren't really looking at heart disease at all. What they found by accident was that, among the 23,000 participants, the men who napped had a 37 percent decrease in deaths from heart disease. (Napping had no effect on women and heart disease.) Why does napping help a man's heart? We don't know for sure, but the researchers think it's because it reduces stress.

Many people wake up from a nap feeling refreshed and full of renewed creativity—so much so that some companies now encourage napping, and even set aside quiet areas for it. So, if you feel the need for a brief snooze in the afternoon, find a comfy spot and sack out. Limit your nap to about 20 to 30 minutes, though. If you sleep any longer, you'll probably go into the deeper stages of sleep. You'll find it hard to wake up and be alert if that happens. Some people find that even 5 or 10 minutes is enough to feel refreshed. I like to take a caffeine nap. Because it takes about 20 to 30 minutes for my afternoon coffee to kick in, I have a cup and then stretch out in my office chair for a nap. The caffeine usually wakes me up in about 20 minutes.

One note of caution here: if you feel the need for long naps, snore while you nap, or have an irresistible urge to nap during the day, these can be signs of underlying health problems. Check with your doctor if you feel you're napping too much or having problem daytime sleepiness.

You Are Getting Sleepy ...

We all have the occasional bad night in which we have trouble getting enough sleep to feel energetic the next day. When "bad nights" happen more than just now and then, however, they can become very disruptive. According to the National Institutes of Health, insomnia and other sleep disorders affect at least 40 million Americans and account for some $16 billion in medical costs every year.[86] And that's not counting the cost of lost work time and other factors, such as accidents caused by drowsiness.

Insomnia is defined as having trouble falling asleep or staying asleep, or having unrefreshing sleep even though you had enough sleep time. Occasional insomnia happens to almost everyone. It's often brought on by worry about work, school, or family, or by stressful events. Minor aches and pains also can cause occasional insomnia. Chronic insomnia is defined as having sleep trouble at least three nights a week for at least one month. About 10 percent of all adults have chronic insomnia. It's more common in women than men, and the incidence goes up in both sexes with age. There are lots of causes of chronic insomnia, but they mostly fall into these four main categories:

- Anxiety, depression, or a physical disease such as arthritis or asthma. Symptoms of many health problems often are worse at night, making it hard to fall asleep or stay asleep.
- Prescription and over-the-counter medications that disrupt sleep, such as antihistamines and steroids
- Sleep-disrupting behavior, such as drinking alcohol; exercising too close to bedtime; or schedule changes from shift work, jet lag, or other causes
- Another sleep disorder, such as sleep apnea or restless legs syndrome (a condition that causes unpleasant tingling or prickling sensations in the legs that can only be relieved by massage or movement)

Fortunately, you can take a lot of self-help steps to relieve insomnia. I've already mentioned some basic sleep hygiene steps that will help you settle down to sleep. Now it's time to look at some simple, commonsense steps that can deal with the specific issues that are the most common causes of insomnia.

First, discuss your physical health and any medications you take with your doctor. It's possible that you may need a mild pain reliever to help with arthritis, for instance. On the other hand, maybe you don't really need some of the medications you are taking. If you feel a specific medication is causing sleeplessness, your doctor may be able to switch you to another. If not, maybe it would be better to take the medication in the morning. Also talk with your doctor about the possibility that sleep apnea, restless legs syndrome, or a neurological problem, such as Parkinson's disease, could be causing your insomnia.

If you and your doctor rule out physical causes of insomnia, that still leaves two big factors: stress and sleep-schedule disruption. Here's where self-help can really pay off.

How to Fall Asleep

Nothing could be simpler than just falling asleep, right? Wrong—at least for the millions of people who find themselves tossing and turning every night, unable to shut off their brains long enough to relax and sleep. That used to be a problem for me, too. Fortunately, I've learned some easy relaxation techniques that are very effective, especially if you combine them with the good sleep practices I discussed earlier in this chapter. Ever wonder how dogs and cats fall asleep so easily? They seem to have a "snooze-on-demand" button. Ever wonder how a baby can, well, sleep like a baby?

Babies, dogs, cats, turtles, birds, elephants, and cows never suffer from insomnia. And they all have one thing in common: unlike you and me, they don't have a "verbal chatterbox" that keeps them up at night.

A verbal chatterbox is the language-based voice with which you and I think. I first spoke about the verbal chatterbox in chapter four. It is your verbal chatterbox that chastises you about all the things you've done wrong in the past, reminds you of all your present problems, and frightens you with all of the potential dangers of the future. It reminds you of the things you have to do, the things you've done, and the things you've failed to do.

Your verbal chatterbox is located in your upper brain, or cerebral cortex, as discussed in an earlier chapter. It's a part of the brain that's underdeveloped in babies and lower mammals, and not present at all in other animals. Your verbal chatterbox is responsible for your deep thoughts and emotions. And it only shuts up when you're sleeping.

Imagine how a baby or a dog or cat must think. Surely they have memories and emotions, but they can't truly understand the concepts of past, present, and future. They can't comprehend, "what if," "if only," "I should have." They're not worried about cancer, bills, terrorism, or violence. They don't replay the details of mistakes or joys in their minds. They can't because they don't have a language, and they don't have a verbal chatterbox.

The key to falling asleep is to turn off your verbal chatterbox, clear your mind of the past and future, and concentrate solely on the present (which is being comfortable in bed, with your eyes closed. That's all. Nothing else.).

All sleeping techniques, from counting sheep to prescription drugs, are designed to turn off your verbal chatterbox. Counting sheep does so by shouting over the verbal chatterbox; prescription drugs do it by chemically disabling the chatterbox.

Turning Off Your Verbal Chatterbox

Your verbal chatterbox controls most of your waking life. To fall asleep, you must use self-control to turn it off. This means you must totally clear your mind of all thoughts—a difficult process that many people have never done. But like any other difficult process, it becomes easier and easier with practice.

Prepare yourself and your environment for sleep as outlined earlier in this chapter. Get comfortable and close your eyes. Imagine a dot floating about two feet in front of your eyes. The dot is slightly up above your forehead. Concentrate on that dot. Any thought, any chatter that comes into your head must be discarded. Move your closed eyes to the periphery, discard the thought, and refocus on the dot. Keep focusing on the dot and keep clearing your mind until you fall asleep.

Before I first tried this technique more than 20 years ago, I thought that keeping your mind blank was impossible. I didn't realize at that time that my verbal chatterbox had an on-off switch. As you engage this technique, you will go through some interesting—and not unpleasant—stages.

As you clear your mind and begin to fall asleep, you will have tiny "dreamette" episodes. You're not quite asleep, yet you are not quite awake. Reality will blur as a friend (who isn't there) talks to you; you might find yourself on vacation somewhere else. Even if you never fully fall into a deep sleep, the dreamettes are quite relaxing.

Here is the key: you are not done with this exercise until you have fallen asleep. Don't give up!

If you read other conventional wisdom about falling asleep, you'll find the advice saying that if you don't fall asleep within 20 minutes, you should get up and walk around or do something else. At the same time, they also say not to watch the clock. That's a contradiction right there! How will you know when 20 minutes have gone by if you're not watching the clock? And if you are, how will you relax and fall asleep?

The key is not to give up. Keep your eyes on the dot and your mind clear until you fall asleep. Control your breathing. Breathe in and out, slowly and deeply, and concentrate on the dot.

You may be thinking, "What if I never fall asleep?" Well, you might not. But you'll still have rested and relaxed, which is better than getting up and walking around, watching TV, or reading.

The real answer is that you *will* fall asleep—eventually. This technique will *always* work if you don't give up. And practice makes perfect. Even the best athletes and musicians need constant practice to achieve and perfect their skills. If you consistently use this technique, you'll soon learn to fall asleep quickly and easily.

Natural Sleep Aids

All sorts of nonprescription sleep aids fill the shelves of drugstores. Most of them work—at least sort of—but they come with long lists of side effects and warnings; they also may be addictive. I prefer natural herbs, such as valerian, as sleep aids. In addition, two supplements—5-HTP (a form of tryptophan) and melatonin—can be effective. The good thing about herbs and these supplements is that they don't drug you to sleep. You sleep more naturally and wake up without grogginess. Remember, though, that these sleeping aids are not magic. They will work best if combined with the sleeping technique outlined above.

Herbal sleep aids. The most widely recommended herbal sleep aid is valerian. It's a mild sedative that's generally safe for most people.

It also doesn't interact with other medications. Valerian has one big drawback: it smells bad. Don't even try any sort of valerian tea; instead, use capsules from a reputable manufacturer. The usual dose is 150 mg to 300 mg, but that can vary a lot from person to person. Start with the smallest possible dose and work up to an amount that helps you; take it about half an hour before bedtime.[87] Other herbal sleep remedies include capsules or tea whose ingredients include lemon balm, chamomile, hops, or catnip (it may get cats a little crazy, but it relaxes people). Kava is sometimes recommended as a sleep aid, but this South Pacific herb may not be safe for regular use. Among other problems, it can cause liver damage and may interact with other medications, especially drugs taken for Parkinson's disease.[88]

5-HTP. Your body uses the amino acid tryptophan to make serotonin, a neurotransmitter, and melatonin. Tryptophan is found naturally in many foods, including turkey, peanuts, oranges, bananas, whole grains, cottage cheese, and milk. Serotonin has an effect on your mood; too little serotonin, and you may feel anxious and depressed. Melatonin is the master hormone for sleep. By keeping your tryptophan levels high, you give your body the raw materials to make serotonin and melatonin, which, in turn, can help you sleep. In the 1990s, a manufacturing problem caused tainted batches of tryptophan, and the product was removed from stores. A safe version of tryptophan called 5-HTP is now available. It can be helpful as a sleep aid. The usual dose is 50 mg to 100 mg, taken about an hour before bedtime. If you prefer to eat your tryptophan, try having a snack of high-tryptophan food, such as peanut butter on whole-wheat bread, about an hour before bedtime. [89]

Melatonin. As we age, we make less melatonin. In fact, by the time you're in your late sixties, you may not make much melatonin at all. That could be one reason insomnia problems are more common among older people. Even if you're still making plenty of melatonin, however, it's a useful supplement to help treat insomnia. It's been shown to be especially helpful for the elderly and people who have trouble getting to sleep because of jet lag or shift work. Melatonin supplements are safe and unlikely to interact with any other medication you might be taking. It's hard to define the best dose. Research suggests that a small amount may work as well as a large dose. So, start with the smallest dose—usually 0.5 mg—and slowly increase it until you find the amount that works for you, but don't go above 20 mg a night. Melatonin usually works best if you take it ninety minutes to two hours before bedtime.[90]

CHAPTER 7

Don't Play with Matches

The statistics are frightening: every year in the United States, accidental injuries claim more than 110,000 lives. Some 43,000 deaths are caused by car crashes alone. Accidents of all sorts seriously injure more than 23 million Americans every year—more than 2.5 million in car crashes. The vast majority of these tragic deaths and injuries could easily be avoided with simple, commonsense measures, such as having working smoke detectors in the home.

Your health is another area where common sense can have a major impact. Quit smoking, drink in moderation, get preventive medical care: all are very basic steps that could have major positive impacts on your health.

Even though easy steps for leading a healthier, safer life are readily available, many people fail to take them. One big reason is simple lack of awareness. In this chapter I want to alarm you—literally!

It Was an Accident

Accidents happen, but most of them shouldn't. In fact, about 80 percent of all bad accidents (the kind where someone ends up hurt) are completely avoidable. Ask a person after an accident—assuming he or she can talk—why it happened, and the answer is pretty likely to be that someone did one (or more) of these things:

- Cut corners, took a shortcut, tried to save time, used the wrong tool. Shortcuts and improvisations that cut into safety and cause accidents are counterproductive, to say the least.
- Ignored safety procedures. A few years ago, a repair shop in my town blew up because a mechanic was siphoning gasoline from a car while another mechanic was using a welding torch on it. Gas fumes, a spark, and kaboom! There's a reason for safety procedures and warning labels. Follow them.
- Got distracted. You're perched on a ladder cleaning leaves out of the gutters when your cell phone rings just as your dog starts to chases the mailman. You fumble for the phone, shout at the dog, and fall off the ladder. Focus on the task at hand and remove as many distractions as possible. Distractions, as I'll discuss later, are a major cause of car crashes.
- Thought they knew what they were doing. This is otherwise known as overconfidence. I once nearly cut off my thumb because I thought I already knew how to use a hedge trimmer. Read the manual first—it's much harder to hold with a big bandage on your thumb.
- Accidents are the fifth-leading cause of death in America, just after chronic lung disease and before complications of diabetes. More than 112,000 people die from unintentional injuries every year. Here's the top ten countdown from the CDC on what causes fatal accidents:
- Machinery—about 350 people a year, mostly on farms
- Medical and surgical complications—about 500 people a year
- Poisoning by gases—about 700 people a year, mostly by carbon monoxide (CO) poisoning
- Firearms—about 1,500 people a year, mostly young men between the ages of 14 and 25
- Suffocation—about 3,300 people a year, usually by choking on food
- Fires and burns—about 3,700 people a year

- Drowning—about 4,000 people a year
- Poisoning by solids and liquids—about 8,600 people a year in a wide variety of ways, including drug overdoses
- Falls—nearly 15,000 people a year and rising
- Car crashes—the top cause of accidental death by a huge margin, these claim more than 43,000 lives a year

The amazing—and tragic—part of this list is that almost all those deaths are avoidable.

On the Road Again

On a typical Memorial Day weekend in America, about 4,000 people are killed or injured in car crashes. About half those crashes involve alcohol; another substantial portion involve drowsy drivers. About a third of the deaths could have been prevented if seat belts had been used. Most tragically of all, almost all the deaths and injuries could have been prevented with simple precautions and some common sense.

Drunk driving. The dangers of drinking and driving are so well known that I won't discuss them here. Instead, I'll scare you. According to the CDC, of all the people killed in car crashes in recent years, more than 17,000 of them had alcohol in their systems. That's roughly 40 percent of all car crash fatalities. Another way to look at that: more than 17,000 needless deaths each year. Or, an alcohol-related car crash kills someone every 31 minutes. Or, someone gets hurt in an alcohol-related car crash every two minutes. The annual cost of alcohol-related crashes is about $51 billion.[91]

With these statistics, I'm not just hoping to scare you into not drinking and driving. I'm hoping to raise your awareness of the problem so that you'll watch out for impaired drivers and avoid them on the road—and report them to the police when possible. Drivers who straddle the center line, weave, drive without lights at night, or make wider than normal turns or abrupt stops at traffic signals are likely to be impaired.

In the mid-1970s, alcohol was a much greater factor in car crashes—more than 60 percent of traffic deaths involved alcohol. Stricter laws and firmer enforcement have brought the number down to 40 percent of fatalities, which proves that getting drunk drivers off the road is the surest way to lessen the carnage. Despite that, there are still plenty of drunks on the road. They're most likely to be driving dangerously between 2:00 and 3:00 AM on Sunday morning, after the bars close on Saturday night partiers. If you can, stay off the road at this time when you are 20 times more likely to be in a fatal crash than at other times of day or night.[92]

Drowsy driving. We all know not to drink and drive, but far too many of us aren't aware of the risks of drowsy driving. Like drunk driving, it's both dangerous and preventable. According to the National Highway Traffic Safety Administration, driver fatigue is the direct cause of at least 100,000 car crashes every year, leading to some 1,500 deaths, 71,000 injuries, and $12.5 billion in cost. These numbers are probably way too low, because the NHTSA also estimates that about a million crashes are caused each year by driver inattention—and inattention is often a side effect of driver fatigue.

One problem with drowsy driving is that you can start the trip feeling alert and energetic, and not notice as drowsiness sets in. Watch out for these warning signs:

- Difficulty focusing your eyes, frequent blinking, heavy eyelids
- Drifting from your lane, swerving, tailgating, hitting rumble strips
- Head nodding
- Yawning frequently
- Trouble remembering the last few miles you drove
- Missing your exit, not noticing traffic signs

Blaring the radio, turning up the air conditioning, or opening the window to let in cold air probably won't help. Caffeine can help in the short run, but if you're short of sleep or really drowsy, it won't keep you alert enough to drive. If you or your passengers notice that you're nodding off behind the wheel, the one thing that will help for sure is to get off the road as quickly and safely as possible. Switch drivers if you can; if not, stop driving and take a 15- to 20-minute nap.

The best defense: avoid drowsy-driving from the start. Follow these safe-travel tips:

- Get a good nights' sleep before you start your trip.
- On long trips, take a break every two hours or one hundred miles. Get out of the car and stretch, then walk around a little and get some fresh air.
- Avoid driving between midnight and 7:00 AM—that's when you're most likely to be too sleepy to drive safely
- Avoid alcohol and any medications—over-the-counter and prescription—that make you drowsy or affect your driving ability. Alcohol will have a more powerful effect on you if you're already sleep deprived.

Most important of all: allow plenty of time to get to your destination. If you're rushed, you'll be less likely to put all the other advice into practice.

Wear your seat belt. Let me repeat that: wear your seat belt. This is the biggest no-brainer of all when it comes to driving safety. Yet about 20 percent of drivers at any given time aren't buckled up. Seat belts save lives—there's no excuse for not using them. My family has always been fanatical about seat belt. When my kids were young and were playing "school bus," the first thing they did was to fasten their imaginary seat belts. They would no sooner ride in a car without wearing a seat belt than go to school without wearing clothing.

As a parent, you need to set a good example by always wearing your seat belt. Be sure everyone, yourself included, is belted in correctly before turning on the engine.

Use child restraints properly. Child safety seats have dramatically reduced injuries and deaths in car crashes. Even so, parents are moving children out of safety seats and booster seats before it's safe to do so. In general, children under the age of eight need child restraints, not adult seat belts. Until children reach age one, they should ride in rear-facing safety seats. Children who are at least one year old and weigh at least 20 pounds can ride in forward-facing safety seats. Children should start using a booster seat when they outgrow their child safety seats, usually when they weigh about 40 pounds. They should continue using booster seats until they get to be four feet nine inches tall—the height at which standard lap and shoulder belts fit properly.

Unfortunately, child safety seats and booster seats often are installed incorrectly. One study found that 72 percent of child restraint systems weren't being used properly.[93] Every brand of car safety seat or booster seat is different. Read the instructions carefully that come with the seat, and hold onto them for future reference. Also check your car manual for instructions on installing safety seats.

Some other precautions for children and cars:

- No child under the age of 13 should ride in the front seat. This avoids air-bag injuries.
- Don't leave a child alone in a car. The temperature inside a closed car can reach a deadly level in just minutes. In addition, children left alone in cars can get caught in power windows, sunroofs, and accessories. They've even been known to knock a car into gear and set it in motion.
- Don't leave a child alone near a car. It's all too easy for a driver to back over a child.

Driving to distraction. A major cause of car crashes is distraction—things that take your attention and concentration away from driving. The National Highway Traffic Safety Administration (NHTSA) says that driver distraction accounts for more 1.5 million police-reported crashes every year. More than 7 million drivers who have been involved in crashes say that distractions were the cause.

Here's a list of the top driving distractions, courtesy of the NHTSA:

- Fiddling with the radio, CD player, or tape deck
- Children
- Pets
- Eating
- Drinking
- Smoking
- Cell phones
- Personal grooming

Some simple commonsense steps could reduce your chances of being distracted by any of the above

- Instead of fiddling with the sound system, ask a passenger to change the CDs, or use a multiple CD changer; use radio presets for your favorite stations.
- If you simply must talk on your cell phone while driving, use a hands-free system and keep the conversation short. (In many states using a hand-held cell phone while driving is now illegal.)
- If you absolutely must eat while driving, select finger foods in small pieces that are easy to hold. Avoid foods that will dribble, drip, or leak. Ditto for drinking while driving—use a travel cup or a go-cup with a straw. Even better, avoid the drive-through completely. Take a break and eat at a table instead.
- Children, even when safely buckled up in the back seat, often demand your attention. The natural parent thing to do is to turn around and glance at them. Instead, let them know that you really love them, and that their safety demands that you

watch the road. "I'm sorry, honey," I used to say to my daughter. "Daddy's driving, and I can't look now. I love you, though, and we can just talk."

- As for smoking and personal grooming while driving, I have just one simple word of advice: Don't.

Older drivers. Driving safely can be a real problem for many older adults—but giving up the mobility and independence of a car can be just as big a problem. Fortunately, with some adjustments, many older adults can continue to drive. People with poor night vision, for instance, can still drive safely during the day. Other adjustments, such as hand controls or wide mirrors, can make driving easier and safer for people with vision or mobility problems. Talk to your doctor about ways to stay behind the wheel safely. In some cases, physical or occupational therapy can improve the driving ability of older adults. So can special driving courses designed for older adults—and if you take one, you also might get a discount on your auto insurance. Check with your local AAA office or AARP for driver-safety refresher courses in your area.

Teen drivers. In the United States, traffic accidents cause two out of every five deaths for teens between the ages of 15 and 19. Worldwide, traffic accidents are the leading cause of death for that age range. As the parent of teenagers, those are statistics that really scare me. But no matter how much I'd like to keep my teenagers out of cars until they're 30, I know that's not really possible. Instead, I take the tough-dad approach and set firm rules about driving—and firm guidelines about what will happen if any of those rules are broken. My kids will tell you I'm an unreasonable ogre, but I disagree—at least about the unreasonable part. We know from the NHTSA and other sources that, for example, teen drivers are more likely to have fatal crashes when other teenagers are in the car. The more teen passengers, the greater the risk. We watch this very carefully at our home. For new drivers, night driving is a high-risk activity. The nighttime fatal crash rate for 16-year-olds is about twice as high as the daytime rate. That's why many states have graduated driver-licensing laws that restrict young drivers from nighttime driving. If you don't live in a state with graduated laws, you'll have to be firm about restricting your teen's nighttime driving. That's because most fatal nighttime crashes happen between 9:00 PM and midnight.

Other rules about teen driving almost go without saying (but say them anyway—and enforce them). Teens should always wear their seat belts, always drive at safe speeds, and never drink and drive. They also should never ride with anyone who ignores these rules. I can remember vividly a talk my fifth grade teacher, Miss Britton, gave us: "I don't care if you only have a dime in your pocket. If you are in a car with someone who is not driving safely, then tell them to pull over, and get out!" That was before cell phones! Today, there is no reason for your children—or anyone—to be a passenger in a car where the driver is drunk or driving in an unsafe manner. My children know that they can call me and I will come and pick them up, any time, any place—no questions asked.

Car maintenance. When we think of the causes of car crashes, the things that come to mind most often are alcohol, excess speed, bad weather, and on the like. We don't usually think about the car itself. But in fact, neglected car maintenance is a big cause of accidents. It's your responsibility to keep your vehicle in good condition.

Tire care tops the list. Underinflated tires can lead to dangerous blowouts. Not only that, driving with underinflated tires is like driving with the parking brake on. It will worsen your gas mileage by about one to two miles per gallon. It costs nothing to check your tire pressure, and inflating the tire to the proper pressure (it's marked on the tire) usually costs just a quarter at any gas station. Bald tires or tires with uneven tread wear also are dangerous, especially on wet or slippery roads.

Another simple, inexpensive maintenance step: make sure your wipers work. Change the blades every six months, preferably in the spring and fall. While you're at it, fill up the washer fluid reservoir.

Walking and Biking Safely

Some of the closest calls I've had in traffic weren't while I was behind the wheel—they were while I was walking, running, or riding a bike. Rule number one for safety in those cases: be alert. There are a lot of bad drivers out there.

If you're out walking, running, or jogging, follow these basic rules:

- If there's a sidewalk, use it.
- If you must walk in the roadway, do so facing the traffic. And don't assume that all drivers will remember that pedestrians have the right of way.
- Dress correctly. Wear light-colored or reflective clothing that can be seen in low light or at night.
- Walk with a buddy. It's safer (and more fun!). If you go out by yourself, tell someone where you're going and approximately when you'll return.
- Stay safe. Leave valuables at home, vary your routes, and carry a cell phone and ID.
- Bike riders face even more hazards than walkers and runners, including the danger of crashing your bike on your own. So, always wear your bike helmet, but remember that a helmet won't keep you from crashing or being hit by a car. You need your common sense for protection against accidents.

As with walking and running, follow these basic safety rules:

- Use bike paths and bike lanes whenever possible, even when it means a less direct route. Streets with bike lanes are significantly safer than streets without them.[94]
- Stay to the right in bike lanes so faster cyclists can easily pass you.
- Don't ride on sidewalks. It's generally not legal. Plus, a lot of

bike accidents happen when a rider moves off the sidewalk into the street.

- If you ride in the street, you must follow the same traffic rules as vehicles, including signaling turns, stopping for lights, and so on.

- Think of yourself as driving a self-propelled car rather than riding a bike, and equip your bike accordingly. Your car has headlights, red rear lights, a horn, and a rearview mirror—and so should your bike. A lot of bike riders like helmet-mounted headlights, because they can look right at a driver and be sure the driver sees them. As for a rearview mirror, try a small one that attaches to your helmet instead of one that fits on the bike.

- If you must ride in traffic, ride like a driver. As a driver, you wouldn't pull up in the parking lane on the right (the blind side) of another car at a stoplight. Why? Because when the light changes, if the other car turns right while you're trying to go straight ahead, you'll get clobbered. Despite the obvious dangers of this, I see bike riders do it all the time. Stay out of the blind spot by riding as far to the left as possible, and passing on the left.

- Use your common sense and ride safely at all times, not just when sharing the road. Only about 10 percent of bike accidents involve motor vehicles.

Children on bikes are especially at risk of an accident. More children end up in the emergency room for a bike-related crash or fall than for any other sports-related injury.[95] Several times a year, a child comes into my office with bleeding lips and cracked teeth. I always look at him and ask, "How fast were you riding your bicycle?" "How did you know?" is the invariable answer.

Establish rules, based on your children's abilities, for when and where they can ride their bikes. As a general rule, children under the age of 10 aren't mature enough to ride safely in the street, and no young child should be riding at night. Make sure that your children's bikes are in good condition and are appropriate for each child's size and ability. Children may be even more prone than adults to think that wearing a helmet is some sort of magical protection against an accident. Strongly emphasize to your children that the helmet won't keep an accident from happening—only they can do that, by riding safely.

Falling for Safety

There's a good chance that you're just one step away from becoming another safety statistic. Falls in the home are a major source of injury and death. In fact, according to the CDC, accidental falls are by far the leading cause of home injuries and deaths. Falls at home account for more than 5 million injuries and nearly 6,000 deaths every year.[96]

As with most other home hazards, commonsense steps can prevent falls. The first and most important step is to do a fall-proofing walkthrough of your home. Make sure these safety features are in place:

- All stairs and steps should have a secure banister or handrail.
- Porches, stairwells, and hallways should be well lit.
- Bathrooms, stairs, and halls should have nightlights.
- Stairs, steps, landings, hallways, and other high-traffic areas should be free of clutter, small end tables, extension and electrical cords, phone cords, and anything else that could trip someone.
- Toys should not be left on steps or landings. Use safety gates at the top and bottom of stairs to protect young children.
- Use a nonslip mat or safety strips in the bathtub and shower. Use a nonskid bath mat.
- Install grab bars in tubs and showers, and near the toilet.
- Put window guards on upper windows to keep children (and pets) from falling out.

- Keep the floor clean and free of clutter. Clean up spills promptly.
- Use a rug liner for throw rugs, or choose rugs with nonskid backing.
- Use a sturdy stepstool if you need to reach items in high places. Never use a chair or kitchen bar stool.
- Use ladders safely. Make sure the ladder is set solidly on a firm, level surface, and set the ladder locks before climbing. Don't sit or stand on the top rung or shelf—it's not designed to carry your weight.

Medications that cause drowsiness, weakness, or dizziness are a major cause of dangerous falls for older adults. Discuss your medications with your doctor. You might be able to reduce your risk by changing the dosage or the medication.

Safe at Home

I admit it—I'm a nut for home safety. It comes in part from my experience as a dentist. I've seen many a tooth that was damaged in a home accident that could easily have been avoided. If you don't want bills from people like me, be careful at home!

Fire safety. Every year some 3,700 Americans die in fires, and some 20,000 are injured. The vast majority of fires occur in the home—and most of them are completely avoidable with some common sense precautions and planning.

- Have at least one working smoke alarm. A smoke alarm doubles your chance of surviving a home fire. They're inexpensive, readily available at the supermarket, and easy to install. There's simply no excuse for not having at least one on every level of your home. Of course, a smoke alarm doesn't do any good if the batteries are dead or have been removed. Test your smoke alarms every month and replace the batteries at least once a year. If your alarm goes off a lot because of smoke from cooking, try moving it to a different location, improving ventilation in your kitchen, and learning to cook better! Whatever you do, *don't take the batteries out of the smoke alarm.*

- Keep several fire extinguishers throughout your home in strategic places—especially the kitchen—and be sure that everyone knows how to use them. Check extinguishers periodically and replace any that have lost pressure.

- Prevent electrical fires. Don't overload outlets or extension cords. Repair or replace any electrical items that sputter, spark, overheat, short out, or give off a smell of burning insulation.

- Be careful with space heaters. Keep anything combustible (blankets, paper, towels, and so on) at least three feet away from portable heaters. Don't use kerosene heaters indoors.

- Don't leave cooking food unattended. Unattended cooking can lead to something much worse than just burned food: it could burn down your house. Thirty percent of home fires—some 50,000 fires a year—start in the kitchen. Of those, most involve someone not paying attention to something cooking on the stovetop.

- Keep fires in the fireplace. Use fire screens, and have your chimney cleaned once a year. Don't use gasoline or other accelerants to start a fireplace fire.

- Don't play with matches. Young children, especially those under the age of five, are naturally curious about fire—to the point where children accidentally set over 20,000 house fires annually.[97] Keep matches and lighters away from children. Careless smoking is another major cause of house fires. Be very careful with matches and lighters, and with lit cigarettes, cigars, and pipes.

- Plan your escape. If a fire does occur, a good escape plan can save you and your family. Plan and practice an escape plan from every room of your house. Get out first, then call for help! When leaving a burning room, stay low to the floor. Feel all doors first, and don't open any that feel hot. Preplan a safe location where everyone can meet after escaping.

Carbon monoxide dangers. The risk of CO poisoning is often overlooked. You can't see or smell CO, but at high levels, it can kill you in just minutes. It's responsible for more than 100,000 poisonings and 500 deaths in the United States each year.

Carbon monoxide is a gas produced whenever any fuel is burned, including oil, natural gas, propane, wood, charcoal, gasoline, and kerosene. That means your furnace, gas range, fireplace, kerosene heater, and car all can be sources of CO. If everything is maintained and used properly, of course, the likelihood of CO poisoning is low. Unfortunately, life is rarely that simple, and sometimes things go wrong through negligence or an accident. Every year, hundreds of people die accidentally from CO poisoning caused by malfunctioning appliances and idling cars. Many more are injured.

The symptoms of CO poisoning are hard to spot. At moderate levels of exposure, you might get a severe headache, become dizzy, confused, nauseated, or faint. You can even die if you're exposed to moderate levels for a long time. Low levels of CO cause shortness of breath, mild nausea, and mild headaches. These are symptoms of lots of other common things, such as the flu, so you might not realize CO is the culprit.

If you have symptoms that might be caused by CO poisoning, don't ignore them—particularly if more than one person in the house is having symptoms. You must act at once to prevent loss of consciousness and death. Get fresh air *immediately*. Open all the doors and windows, turn off whatever device is the source of the CO (such as the oven or furnace), and leave the house at once. Go straight to an emergency room and tell the staff you suspect CO poisoning.

Prevention is the key to avoiding CO poisoning. Have all your fuel-burning appliances inspected once a year. That means checking oil and gas furnaces, gas water heaters, gas ranges and ovens, gas dryers, gas or kerosene space heaters, fireplaces, and wood stoves. Be certain that all flues and chimneys are connected, in good repair, and not blocked in any way.

Idling cars are a major source of CO poisoning, especially when the car runs in a closed garage. Even if the garage door is open, the fumes can build up very quickly and enter the living areas of the house. If you want to warm up the car, pull out into the driveway and leave it running there—with the garage door closed. Similarly, don't use a gasoline-powered engine in an enclosed or unventilated place.

Other common sources of CO problems are using a gas oven to heat your home, using a gas or charcoal grill indoors (don't even use one in the garage, no matter how much you want to barbecue on a rainy day), and using gas or kerosene space heaters in unventilated spaces.

I strongly recommend a CO alarm for your home—and so do government agencies, including the Environmental Protection Agency and the U.S. Consumer Product Safety Commission. A CO detector isn't a replacement for proper use and maintenance of your appliances and car, but it can save your life. Choose a reliable model with long-lasting batteries and install it properly—preferably high up on a wall. Make sure that the model you purchase is UL certified. If the alarm does go off, make sure it's the CO detector and not your smoke alarm.

I had some dear family friends who were killed by CO. He was a physician; she was a dentist. They were intelligent and well educated, but they did not have a CO detector. Both parents and their young daughter were killed by CO, leaving their other two children orphaned.

Radon risks. Another home-safety device to consider is a radon detector. It's a little less of a no-brainer than a smoke alarm or CO detector, but you may still need one.

Radon is a cancer-causing radioactive gas. It's invisible and odorless, but it causes about 21,000 deaths from lung cancer every year—even among nonsmokers. That's *seven times* as many people as the number who die every year from home fires. In fact, radon is second only to smoking as the leading cause of lung cancer in the United States.[98]

Radon occurs naturally all over the country as a result of the breakdown of uranium in soil, rock, and water. Radon can get into any kind of building; today, about one in fifteen homes has a high indoor radon level. That makes home the place where you're most likely to get the greatest exposure.

The only way to know for sure if radon is in your home is to test for it. Even if your neighbor's house is radon-free, yours might not be. Testing is simple, inexpensive, and quick. There are two basic approaches:

- Short-term testing. A radon-detecting device from an inexpensive test kit stays in your home for anywhere from a few days to a few months. Radon levels can vary from day to day and season to season, but a short-term test can still give you an idea of whether radon is present at dangerous levels.
- Long-term testing. This is much like short-term testing, but the detector stays in place for more than 90 days. A long-term test is a good way to get an accurate idea of your home's year-round radon level.

On average, indoor radon levels are around 1.3 pico curies per liter (pCi/L). A reading of above 4.0 pCi/L would be considered dangerous. Fortunately, radon-reduction systems work pretty well and usually aren't too expensive. Even very high radon levels can be lowered to acceptable levels. This isn't a do-it-yourself project, though. Find a qualified specialist by checking with your state radon office; look in the blue pages of your phone book or call your state environmental protection agency. Newer houses are usually built to be radon resistant, but it's still important to check.

Common Sense Steps for a Safer Home

Making your home a safer place is usually just a matter of simple, inexpensive, commonsense steps. Take scalding injuries, for instance. Every year, about 3,800 people are injured by tap water that's too hot. Keeping your home's hot-water thermostat at no more than 120°F can prevent this problem. (If the thermostat doesn't have numbers, 120°F is usually about the middle of the dial, or just below.) Checking the hot-water temperature on your water heater, and lowering it if necessary, is something you might be able to do yourself (consult your owner's manual). If not, call the relevant service company; they may do it for you for free. For electric or gas hot-water heaters, call your local electric or gas company; for an on-line system routed from your oil furnace, call your local fuel supplier. You'll make your home safer and also save on fuel expenses—two benefits for little or no cost.

Kitchen Safety

The kitchen is always the most popular room in the house—and it can be the most dangerous, as well. Aside from the fire danger I mentioned earlier, the kitchen is full of ways for people to get burned, cut, bruised, and poisoned. Here's a really important place to use your common sense.

- Never leave unattended food cooking on the stove or in the oven.
- Keep things that can burn—such as towels, plastic bags, and curtains—at least three feet away from the range.
- Use caution with hot foods and beverages. Always wear oven mitts, and don't lift hot, heavy objects (a large pot full of boiling water) that weigh too much for you.
- Childproof the kitchen. Keep small children and pets away from the range. Use childproof covers on the range knobs. Turn pot handles toward the back of the range, and use the back

burners whenever possible—this prevents children from pulling over a hot pan. Keep small children out of kitchen cabinets and drawers. The cabinet under the sink is the traditional place to store cleaning supplies and other household chemicals—all of which can be very dangerous for small children. Ditto for drawers full of knives and other sharp implements. For this reason, use childproof latches on all cabinet doors and drawers.

Poison Prevention

Accidental poisonings are a leading cause of injury in the home.[99] It's surprisingly easy to get poisoned in your own house. I've already mentioned the problem of CO poisoning, but there are other poison hazards as well. Small children are especially at risk since they will put *anything* in their mouths, even if it's something that (to an adult) obviously tastes terrible. So, in addition to childproofing the kitchen, you also must childproof the rest of the house:

- Take all medicines and medical supplies out of handbags, pockets, drawers, and anyplace else a small child can reach.
- Store all medicines, vitamins, and supplements in a cabinet or drawer with a child-safety lock. Cosmetics, too—they can be dangerous to small children.
- Pick up any dropped pills so children and pets can't get them. A single acetaminophen (Tylenol) tablet can kill a cat.
- Discard old medicines by flushing them away. Or mix them with something unpalatable, such as used coffee grounds, and throw them out.
- Be extra careful with any item labeled with "Caution," "Warning," or "Danger." Store the item in a childproof cabinet or drawer.
- Store gasoline, antifreeze, pool chemicals, pesticides, fertilizers, and all other dangerous products in a safe, childproof place in

the garage or shed. Leave them in their original containers with the original labels. Clean up any spills immediately. Check with your local government or trash collection service for ways to safely discard unwanted products.

- If you suspect poisoning, immediately call 911 or the national poison control hotline at 1-800-222-1222.

Electrical Safety

Our homes are so filled with electrical appliances and tools that we often take the power behind them for granted. Don't. Electrical problems can cause major fires and serious shock injuries. Fortunately, with minimal effort you can keep your home electrically safe.

- Lighting. Use the right light bulb—with the correct wattage—in lamps and light fixtures. There's a label inside every fixture that tells you which bulb is right. To save energy, consider replacing standard light bulbs with compact fluorescent light bulbs. Even thought the compacts give off less heat, don't exceed the wattage for the fixture.
- Electrical systems. Make sure all electrical outlets and switches have covers; install childproof covers on outlets. Any electrical outlet that could come into contact with water (especially in the bathroom or outside) should have a ground fault circuit interrupter (GFCI) to protect you from dangerous shocks. A GFCI can easily be installed by an electrician. Electrical cords should be in good condition; replace any that are damaged. Don't tie or knot cords, and don't set furniture on top of them. If your lights flicker, you smell burning insulation, your circuit breakers trip frequently, or your power goes out a lot, call an electrician at once!
- Appliances. Don't use appliances near water—for example, don't use a hair dryer while you're in the bathtub. Avoid plugging too many appliances into one outlet.

Water Safety

Backyard pools are a wonderful home amenity—but they can also be a home nightmare. I don't mean just keeping the water clean and at the right temperature, or even having to scoop out the occasional drowned chipmunk. I mean the risk of accidental drowning. Don't have a pool? You still have to worry about the risk of accidental drowning. Hidden drowning hazards, especially for young children, are all over your house and yard.

The scariest thing about an accidental drowning is how fast and silently it can happen. Prevention is crucial here, because drowning can happen in any standing water—even a landscape pond or five-gallon bucket.

Several years ago some friends were at my house for a barbecue. The grill was on the patio, just a few yards from the pool. My friends' son, an eight-year-old named Corey, was playing in the pool while we were grilling. We were talking with our backs to the pool. The pool was just yards away, and we were well within earshot; but when we casually turned to face the pool, there was Corey, floating face down and motionless. For a second, we thought he was just playing. There was no thrashing, no screaming, no panic. But he was drowning! I jumped in, pulled him out—and just like in the movies—water shot out of his mouth upon chest compression. Corey was fine, but we all learned a lesson we will never forget: drowning can happen in a flash.

- Swimming pools should be fenced with self-closing gates. This is so important that most municipalities have laws requiring it.
- Supervise everyone in the pool, not just the children. Don't allow anyone to swim alone.
- Keep the area around the pool uncluttered. Put away pool toys and equipment, and store pool chemicals in a safe, childproof place.
- Hot tubs and spas are a major drowning hazard. Always secure the safety cover.
- Large buckets are a drowning hazard for toddlers, who can tum-

ble in head-first. Never leave a full bucket unattended. Empty out buckets and store them upside-down when not in use.

- Toilets are another drowning hazard for toddlers. Leave the lid down and install childproof lid locks.
- Always stay within arm's reach of a baby or small child in the bathtub. Supervise bath time closely, and never leave a child alone. Empty the tub or sink as soon as the bath is over.

Your Health Is Up to You

Lots of people are involved with your health: your family, your doctors, your pharmacist, your insurance company, your employer. With all that involvement and support, however, you still need to be personally responsible for your own health. It's your choice to do things that harm you—and it's also your choice to decide to take steps that will improve your health.

Smoking. My advice about smoking is simple: don't. The evidence that tobacco kills people is crystal clear. So is the evidence that even if tobacco doesn't kill you directly, through lung cancer or emphysema, it will cause other health problems. And those will kill you either directly, or by contributing to your early demise. Even worse, your secondhand smoke will harm those around you, especially your children. In fact, every year spent in a home with smokers causes more than 750,000 middle ear infections in children, and at least 150,000 lung infections in babies.[100] There's no safe level of exposure to tobacco smoke for anyone.

The question isn't really *if* you should stop smoking. You should. It also isn't *when*. Quit now. The real question is *how*, because it's very difficult to give up tobacco.

I can't say I'm speaking from firsthand experience, but because smoking is really, really bad for your oral health, I do have a lot of experience in helping my patients quit. I've learned a great deal from them over the years about what helps and what doesn't. The most important thing I've learned is that it often takes at least two tries before tobacco is out of your life for good. After all, nicotine is an addictive drug; for some people, it can be as addictive as cocaine.[101]

When your brain stops getting the nicotine it craves, it sends out desperate messages that are almost impossible to ignore. And your body goes through very real, very difficult withdrawal symptoms that may lead you to give up. But, if you learn some techniques for dealing with cravings, you can overcome them. The hardest part is hanging in there for the first few days. Once you get past those first days without tobacco, your cravings will probably diminish quite a bit.

It may help you to find something to do with your hands and mouth. I suggest individually wrapped hard candies or chewing gum (sugar-free, please). Whenever you want a cigarette, the act of unwrapping the candy or gum and then chewing on it can make a good substitute. I had a patient who was able to quit by substituting shelled peanuts for cigarettes. Shelling the peanuts gave him something to do with his hands for as long as it took for the cigarette urge to pass. Because peanuts are a healthy food choice, he also was able to avoid the weight gain that often happens when people stop smoking and substitute food for cigarettes. (By the way, studies show that weight gain from quitting smoking is rarely more than 10 pounds.[102] Being a few pounds heavier is still a heck of a lot better than smoking.) Or try eating crunchy, healthy foods, such as carrots and celery sticks. All that chewing may help reduce cravings by keeping your mouth busy like a cigarette does. Another technique that I like a lot as a dentist is brushing your teeth immediately after eating. I don't know why this helps, but it does!

Over the years I've had patients who were helped by all sorts of anti-smoking programs and techniques. Some found hypnotherapy helpful; others benefited from acupuncture. Some found support through instructor-led group programs; others had "quit buddies" who helped keep them on track. Nicotine replacement products, such as nicotine patches or gum, helped some people, too. But for every patient who found these techniques helpful, there were others who didn't. Will-power alone often isn't enough, even when you're very motivated to quit. If one technique isn't helping you, try another.

Alcohol. I talked briefly about the positive health benefits of alcohol in chapter 4. Alcohol in moderation—meaning one drink a day—can be an effective stress-reliever. Alcohol in moderation also may be good for your heart health, but it's important to keep that in perspective and not use it as a reason to have more than one drink a day.

Drinking may indeed lower the risk of heart disease, especially among women older than age 55. A lot of other factors also may reduce the risk, however: eating a healthy diet, getting regular exercise, not smoking, and maintaining a healthy weight. The benefits of alcohol are pretty minor in comparison. And, there's little evidence that moderate drinking provides any health benefit to younger people.

There's plenty of evidence about the risks of too much alcohol, however. Unfortunately, according to recent surveys from the U.S. National Institute on Alcohol Abuse and Alcoholism, some 30 percent of Americans have alcohol problems at some point. What's an alcohol problem? It's any problem related to alcohol use that may require some type of intervention or treatment. You might be what experts call a "risky drinker." That means you consume alcohol in a way that may pose a real risk of physical or emotional harm to yourself or others, but you're not dependent on alcohol and don't regularly abuse it.

You've probably been hearing about the risks of alcohol use ever since grade school. You already know how dangerous anything beyond moderate alcohol consumption can be. You already know how dangerous it is to drink and drive. But did you know that alcohol is involved in 40 percent of all fatal traffic accidents? And did you know that alcohol-related accidents and health problems cost over $51 billion a year?

What you also may not know is that there is a serious risk of dangerous interactions when you combine alcohol with certain drugs. The list of drugs—both prescription and over-the-counter—that are affected by alcohol is very long. It includes many widely prescribed medications such as Valium, Xanax, Celexa, Lexapro, Prozac, Zoloft, Glucophage, Zantac, Lipitor, and Vicodin. Popular nonprescription painkillers as well as cough, cold, and allergy remedies are especially likely to interact badly with alcohol. For example, Tylenol—touted as a safe nonprescription painkiller—can cause severe liver damage when combined with alcohol.

Many medications—prescription or nonprescription—can cause drowsiness, dizziness, impaired judgment, or worse, just by themselves. Add in alcohol, and you have a prescription for falling asleep at the wheel or just plain falling, with potentially serious consequences. Fortunately, the packaging and labeling of a nonprescription drug will warn you about combining it with alcohol. The drug information that comes with any prescription drug will do the same; plus, the pharmacist will put a warning tag on the container. Take these warnings seriously and discuss any questions you have with your doctor or pharmacist. If in doubt, use your common sense—don't drink and take the drug.

Take care of yourself. Just as precautions can help prevent most accidents, many illnesses can be avoided—or can be caught early enough to be more treatable—through health precautions such as screening tests and vaccinations.

Screening tests find diseases such as cancer early, when they're almost always easier to treat. Most screening tests are simple, painless, quick, and covered by health insurance. The screening tests below are the ones recommended by the Agency for Healthcare Research and Quality, part of the Department of Health and Human Services. They're based on the latest research and clinical practice guidelines, but you don't necessarily need every one of them. Talk with your doctor to decide which ones apply to you, and when and how often you should be tested.

- Obesity. Check your BMI and waist measurement at least once every six months.

- High cholesterol. Current recommendations are to check your cholesterol regularly starting at age 35 if you're a man, and age 45 if you're a woman. Start sooner if you smoke, or if you have diabetes, high blood pressure, or a family history of heart disease.
- High blood pressure. Have your blood pressure checked at least once every two years. High blood pressure means a reading of 140/90 or higher.
- Diabetes. If you have high blood pressure or high cholesterol, you may have diabetes as well. Your doctor can check for it with a simple finger-prick blood test.
- Colorectal cancer. Both men and women should get checked for colorectal cancer beginning at age 50, or earlier if there is a family history of the disease. Your doctor can help you decide which type of screening test is best for you. And OK, a colonoscopy is the exception to screening tests that are quick and easy—but this is a test that really could save your life, so have one if your doctor recommends it.
- Breast cancer. Current recommendations are to have a mammogram every one to two years starting at age 40.
- Cervical cancer. Have a Pap smear done every one to three years if you're between the ages of 21 and 65.
- Prostate cancer. There's no routine screening test for prostate cancer. In fact, there's not a lot of agreement among experts about whether screening for prostate cancer is even effective, much less who should be screened and how often. Right now two tests are widely used: the digital rectal exam (OK, another exception to the painless part of screening), and the prostate-specific antigen (PSA) blood test. The PSA is controversial, because a high result on the test could mean you have cancer—or it could mean that you have some other common problem, such as benign prostatic hyperplasia (enlarged prostate), that isn't

cancer and won't become cancer. Talk with your doctor about this one.

- Depression. Your mental health is just as important as your physical health. If you feel down, sad, or hopeless for more than a couple of weeks, or if you lose interest in the things you used to enjoy, talk with your doctor.

- Osteoporosis. In women, some bone loss is normal after menopause, but too much bone loss leads to thin, brittle bones that break easily. All women should be regularly screened for osteoporosis beginning at age 65. There are lots of good reasons to be screened earlier, however, especially if you experience early or surgical menopause, or if osteoporosis runs in your family. Again, talk with your doctor about what's right for you. And don't forget that older men also can develop osteoporosis, especially if they're smokers.

- Sexually transmitted diseases. Don't be shy—talk to your doctor.

- Abdominal aortic aneurysm. An aneurysm is an abnormally large or swollen blood vessel. An abdominal aortic aneurysm is a swelling in the part of the aorta (the main artery that carries blood from your heart) that lies in your abdomen. Although the condition is rare, it's very dangerous. If the aneurysm bursts, you can bleed to death very quickly. Current guidelines call for a one-time ultrasound screening for adults between the ages of 65 and 75, especially if they have ever smoked.

- Other tests for older adults. If you're older than age 65, talk with your doctor about hearing and vision tests.

- Dental checkups. Have these done regularly (go back to chapter 1 to learn why!).

Although I keep saying "talk with your doctor," you may be able to receive some screening tests through community outreach programs of your local hospital, Red Cross, or other organizations. These programs are convenient and often free or very low cost, so take advantage of them.

Preventing disease. One of the easiest and least expensive medications for preventing heart disease is the simple aspirin tablet. This seems to work less well for women than for men; in addition, some people are aspirin resistant.[103] But overall, aspirin seems to be very effective for many people. If you're older than age 45, ask your doctor whether or not you should take aspirin to prevent heart disease. If you're younger than age 45, but you smoke or have high blood pressure, high cholesterol, or diabetes, talk with your doctor. Aspirin therapy might be appropriate for you, too.

Keeping your immunizations up to date also is an important preventive measure. Have a flu shot every year starting at age 50; if you're younger, ask your doctor whether or not you need the shot. If you're older than age 65, talk with your doctor about having a pneumonia shot; if you're younger, ask your doctor if you need one.

Remember all those vaccine booster shots you got when you were a kid? Well, I hate to tell you this, but grown-ups need booster shots, too. Not only that, your doctor probably won't give you a lollipop afterward. Even so, here are the shots that you need as an adult:

- Varicella (chickenpox). If you've never had chickenpox, or aren't sure if you have, this vaccine is now recommended.
- Herpes zoster. This recently approved vaccine prevents shingles, a painful and debilitating viral illness that is more likely to hit as you get older. It's recommended for all adults older than age 60. Herpes zoster, by the way, is *not* caused by the same virus that causes genital herpes.
- Human papillomavirus (HPV). This vaccine targets four different virus strains that can cause cervical cancer and genital warts. It's recommended for all women aged 11 to 26.
- Tetanus-diphtheria-pertussis (Tdap). Pertussis, or whooping

cough, is a serious bacterial disease that is transmitted by adults to babies and young children. Starting in 2005, Tdap is recommended for all adults aged 64 or younger whose last tetanus-diphtheria booster shot was at least 10 years ago. Unless you've been in an emergency room for a bad gash, a rusty nail through your foot, or something else that needed a tetanus shot, you're probably due for a tetanus booster anyway. Talk with your doctor, especially if you're often in contact with children.

- Measles-mumps-rubella (MMR). Older adults who had these childhood illnesses in the days before vaccines don't need boosters, but younger people who were vaccinated against them do.
- Hepatitis A and hepatitis B. These target the viruses that cause serious liver disease. They're recommended for all adults, but especially for health-care workers, people who work with children, and anyone traveling abroad to less-developed countries.
- Meningococcal. A vaccine that prevents meningitis and other meningococcal diseases, this is strongly recommended for students living in college dorms.

Depending on your age and situation, you probably won't need every shot on this list, but any one of them could prevent a serious or even life-threatening illness. Discuss your vaccine schedule with your doctor to decide which ones are right for you.

Live Better, Live Longer—It's Simple

All of the information in this book could best be summed up by a quote from Mark Twain: "It is better to be careful a hundred times than to get killed once."

Contrary to popular belief, usually people don't just "get sick." Usually accidents don't "just happen." More often than not, disease and accidents can be avoided. Throughout this book, I've demonstrated over and over that simple preventive measures—washing your hands, brushing your teeth, wearing seat belts—can help you to live better and live longer. It's simple, yet many people don't follow these easy guidelines.

It's time to incorporate the suggestions in this book into your daily life. It won't take much time or money. These are habits that can quickly become automatic. Begin today, and you will have lots of tomorrows.

Endnotes

1. National Center for Health Statistics, Faststats Life Expectancy table 7
2. CDC National Center for Health Statistics press release, 5/2/2007
3. Deaths and death rates for leading causes of death: death. Registration states, 1900-1940, Centers for Disease Control
4. Deaths and death rates for leading causes of death: death. Registration states, 1900-1940, Centers for Disease Control
5. National Vital Statistics Reports, Volume 55, Number 19, August 21, 2007
6. Periodontal disease and coronary heart disease: an epidemiological and microbiological study. *New Microbiol.* July 2007
7. Endotoxemia, Immune response to periodontal pathogens, and systemic inflammation associate with incident cardiovascular disease events. *Arterioscler Thromb Vasc Biol.* March 15, 2007
8. Severity of periodontal disease correlates to inflammatory systemic status and independently predicts the presence and angiographic extent of stable coronary artery disease. *J Intern Med.* Jan 16, 2008
9. Periodontal disease and pregnancy outcomes: exposure, risk and intervention. *Best Pract Res Clin Obstet Gynaecol.* June, 2007
10. Clinical and metabolic changes after conventional treatment of type 2 diabetic patients with chronic periodontitis. *J Periodontol,* April, 2006
11. Incidence of Hepatitis A in the United States in the Era of Vaccination. *JAMA* July 13, 2005
12. National Center for Health Statistics, Faststats
13. U.S. Census Bureau Statistical Abstract of the United States: 1999 Page 106
14. Periodontal (Gum) Disease. Causes, Symptoms, and Treatment. NIH Publication No. 06-1142 January 2006
15. Relative Contribution of Caries and Periodontal Disease in Adult Tooth Loss for an HMO Dental Population. *Journal of Public Health Dentistry* September 1995
16. Radiographic measures of chronic periodontitis and carotid artery plaque. *Stroke* March 2005
17. Periodontal Microbiota and carotid intima-media thickness: The oral

infections and vascular disease epidemiology study (INVEST). *Circulation* (J Am Heart Assn) 2005 111;576-582

18. Severity of periodontal disease correlates to inflammatory systemic status and independently predicts the presence and angiographic extent of stable coronary artery disease. *J Int Med* , 2008 Jan 16

19. Treatment of periodontitis and endothelial function. *N Enjg J Med* , 2007 Mar 1;356(9):911-20

20. Periodontal care may improve enodthelial function , *Eur J Intern Med* , 2007 Jul;18(4):295-8

21. Severity of periodontal disease correlates to inflammatory systemic status and independently predicts the presence and angiographic extent of stable coronary artery disease. *J Intern Med.* Jan 16, 2008

22. The effect of improved periodontal health on metabolic control in type 2 diabetes mellitus. *J Clin Periodontol.* , 2005 Mar;32(3):266-72

23. Clinical and metabolic changes after conventional treatment of type 2 diabetic patients with chronic periodontitis. *J Periodontol.* 2006 Apr;77(4):591-8

24. Periodontal therapy may reduce the risk of preterm low birth weight in women with periodontal disease: a randomized controlled trial. *J Periodontol.* 2002 Aug; 73(8):911-24

25. Periodontal therapy reduces the rate of preterm low birth weight in women with pregnancy-associated gingivitis. *J Periodontol.* 2005 Nov; 76 (11 Suppl): 2144-53

26. Treatment of periodontal disease and the risk of preterm birth. *N Engl J Med.* 2006 Nov 2; 355(18):1885-94

27. Effect of periodontal therapy on pregnancy outcome in women affected by periodontitis. *J Periodontol.* 2007 Nov; 78(11):2095-103

28. Periodontal health and adverse pregnancy outcome in 3,576 Turkish women. *J Periodontol* 2007 Vol 78, No 11 2081-94

29. Dentition, oral hygiene, and risk of oral cancer: a case-control study in Beijing, People's Republic of China. *Cancer Causes Control.* 1990 Nov;1(3):235-41

30. Relationship between dental factors and risk of upper aerodigestive tract cancer. *Oral Oncol.* 1998 Jul;34(4):284-91

31. The salivary microbiota as a diagnostic indicator of oral cancer: A descriptive, non-randomized study of cancer-free and oral squamous cell carcinoma subjects. *J Transl Med.* 2005 Jun 29,3(1):27

32. A prospective study of periodontal disease and pancreatic cancer in US male health professionals. *J Natl Cancer Inst.* 2007 Jan 17;99(2):171-5

33. *American Dental Association News,* May 18, 2007

34. USDA National Nutrient Database for Standard Reference

35. Calcium and the risk for periodontal disease. *J Periodontol.* 2000 Jul;71(7):1057-66

36. Dietary vitamin C and the risk for periodontal disease *J Periodontol* 2000 Aug;71(8):1215-23

37. Relationship between salivary melatonin and severity of periodontal disease. *J Periodontol* 2006 Sep;77(9):1533-8

38. Centers for disease control. Clean hands coalition.

39. Food-Related Illness and Death in the United States. *Emerging infectious diseases* CDC Vol5 No5

40. The importance of handwashing for your health. Canadian Health Network

41. MRSA Kills One in 20 Hospital Patients Who Have the Infection. Agency for Healthcare Research and Quality (AHRQ) Oct 25, 2007

42. Physical Barriers May Be More Effective Than Drugs To Prevent Pandemics

43. *ScienceDaily* (Dec. 2, 2007)

44. Many Don't Wash Hands After Using the Bathroom. *The New York Times* September 27, 2005

45. Who washes hands after using the bathroom? *Am J Infect Control.* 1997 Oct;25(5):424-5

46. American Society for Microbiology (ASM) and The Soap and Detergent Association (SDA) Handwashing Survey, Sept. 2007

47. Yves Thomas, head of the National Influenza Research Centre at Geneva University Hospital. Reuters telephone interview, January 2008

48. Food and Drug Administration (FDA) Nonprescription Drugs Advisory Committee meeting by SDA and CTFA issue brief October 20, 2005.

49. Effectiveness of a nonrinse, alcohol-free antiseptic hand wash. *J Am Podiatr Med Assoc.* 2001 Jun;91(6):288-93.

50. Effect of hand sanitizer use on elementary school absenteeism. *Am J Infect Control* Oct;28(5):340-6

51. A randomized, controlled trial of a multifaceted intervention including alcohol-based hand sanitizer and hand-hygiene education to reduce illness transmission in the home. *Pediatrics.* 2005 Sep;116(3):587-94

52. Food-Related Illness and Death in the United States *Emerging Infectious Diseases* Vol5 No5

53. Update on Multi-State Outbreak of *E. coli* O157:H7 Infections From Fresh Spinach. CDC report October 6, 2006 Science News Online Sept 14, 1996

54. Is your desk making you sick? *CNN.com* November 13, 2006

55. A prospective study of weight change and systemic inflammation over 9 y. *Am J Clin Nutr* 2008 Jan;87(1):30-5.

56. Weight status and restaurant availability a multilevel analysis. Am J Prev Med. 2008 Feb;34(2):127-33

57. Double-blind randomised trial of modest salt restriction in older people. *Lancet* 1997 Sep 20;350(9081):850-4
58. Trans fatty acids and coronary heart disease. *N Engl J Med.* 1999 Jun 24;340(25):1994-8
59. Addressing the health benefits and risks, involving vitamin D or skin cancer, of increased sun exposure. Proc Natl Acad Sci USA 2008 Jan 15;105(2):668-73.
60. Job Strain and Risk of Acute Recurrent Coronary Heart Disease Events JAMA October 10, 2007
61. Stress and relapse of breast cancer. BMJ. 1989 February 4; 298(6669): 291–293
62. Stress in the Workplace. American Psychological Association: APA Health Center
63. Effect of social networks on 10 year survival in very old Australians: the Australian longitudinal study of aging Journal of Epidemiology and Community Health 2005;59:574-579
64. National Institute on Alcohol Abuse and Alcoholism No. 16 PH 315 April 1992
65. Alcohol Amount, Not Type -- Wine, Beer, Liquor -- Triggers Breast Cancer. ScienceDaily (Sep. 28, 2007)
66. Physical activity, physical fitness and longevity. Aging 1997 Feb-Apr;9(1-2):2-11.
67. Effects of physical activity on life expectancy with cardiovascular disease. *Arch Intern Med* 2005 Nov 14;165(20):2355-60.
68. Physical activity recommendations and decreased risk of mortality. *Arch Intern Med* 2007 Dec 10;167(22):2453-60.
69. High-intensity strength training in nonagenarians. Effects on skeletal muscle. *JAMA* 1990 Jun 13;263(22):3029-34.
70. Self-efficacy correlates with leg muscle pain during maximal and sub-maximal cycling exercise. *J Pain* 2007 Jul;8(7):583-7.
71. Understanding Dog Owners' Increased Levels of Physical Activity: Results From RESIDE. *American Journal of Public Health* January 2008
72. U.S. Department of Health and Human ServicesNational Institutes of Health. National Institute of Diabetes and Digestive and Kidney Diseases NIH Pub No. 06-5578 January 2006
73. The combined influence of leisure-time physical activity and weekly alcohol intake on fatal ischaemic heart disease and all-cause mortality. *Eur Heart J* 2008 Jan;29(2):204-212.
74. Sleep Disorders and Sleep Deprivation: An Unmet Public Health Problem. Institute of Medicine Report. April 04, 2006
75. SLEEP 2007: the 21st Annual Meeting of the Associated Professional Sleep Societies: Abstract 0089. Presented June 13, 2007.
76. Effect of sleep loss on c-reactive protein an inflammatory marker of car-

diovascular risk. Preventive Cardiology Abstract ACC Current Journal Review Vol 13 Issue 4

77. North American Association for the Study of Obesity (NAASO)'s Annual Scientific Meeting held November 14-18, 2004. Presented by researcher James Gangwisch

78. A Prospective Study of Self-Reported Sleep Duration and Incident Diabetes in Women. *Diabetes Care* 26:380-384, 2003

79. Association of sleep time with diabetes mellitus and impaired glucose tolerance. *Arch Intern Med* 2005 Apr 25;165(8):863-7

80. In Brief: Your Guide to Healthy Sleep. NIH Publication No. 06–5800 April 2006

81. NHTSA Vehicle Safety Rulemaking And Supporting Research Priorities:Calendar Years 2005-2009

82. Sleep and adolescent suicidal behavior. *Sleep* 2004 Nov 1;27(7):1351-8.

83. The relationship of glucose tolerance to sleep disorders and daytime sleepiness. *Diabetes Res Clin Pract.* 2005 Jan;67(1):84-91

84. Who Is At Risk for Sleep Apnea? U.S. Department of Health & Human Services. National Heart, Lung and Blood Institute. Diseases and Conditions Index

85. Siesta in Healthy Adults and Coronary Mortality in the General Population. *Arch Intern Med.* 2007;167:296-301.

86. Brain Basics: Understanding Sleep. National Institutes of Health. National Institute of Neurological Disorders and Stroke. NIH Publication No.06-3440-c May 21, 2007

87. Valerian. National Institutes of Health. Office of Dietary Supplements.

88. Kava-Containing Dietary Supplements May Be Associated With Severe Liver Injury. Consumer Advisory Center for Food Safety and Applied Nutrition, U.S. Food and Drug Administration March 25, 2002

89. Report: Contamination found in L-tryptophan supplement. CNN Interactive August 31, 1998

90. Melatonin. MedlinePlus U.S. National Library of Medicine and the National Institutes of Health.

91. Impaired Driving. Department of Health and Human Services. Centers for Disease Control and Prevention.

92. National Highway Traffic Safety Administration (NHTSA)

93. Child Restraint Use Survey LATCH Use and Misuse. National Technical Information Service, DOT HS 810 679 December 2006

94. Bicycle Lanes Versus Wide Curb Lanes: Operational and Safety Findings and Countermeasure Recommendations Federal Highway Administration FHWA-RD-99-035

95. Consumer Product Safety Commission's Consumer Product Safety Review - Spring, 2000

96. Home Safety Council's State of Home Safety in America. Sept 2004

97. Quiet Disasters: House Fires Destroy Lives Every Day. American Red Cross. In the News. April 6, 2001

98. http://www.epa.gov/radon/healthrisks.html. Health Risks Exposure to Radon Causes Lung Cancer In Non-smokers and Smokers Alike U.S. Environmental Protection Agency

99. Home Safety Council's State of Home Safety in America. Sept 2004

100. Environmental tobacco smoke and middle ear disease in preschool-age children. *Arch Pediatr Adolesc Med.* 1998 Feb;152(2):127-33

101. Surgeon General Asserts Smoking Is an Addiction. *The New York Times* May 17, 1988

102. Dr. Michael Fiore, director of the Center for Tobacco Research and Intervention and professor of medicine at the University of Wisconsin Medical School. . http://www.surgeongeneral.gov/tobacco/fiore.htm

103. Aspirin "resistance" and risk of cardiovascular morbidity: systematic review and meta-analysis. *BMJ*, Jan 2008; 336: 195 – 198

Addendum

Bibliography for Chapter 1

Accarini R, Periodontal disease as a potential risk factor for acute coronary syndromes, Arq Bras Cardiol, 2006 Nov;87(5):592-6

Amabile N, Severity of periodontal disease correlates to inflammatory systemic status and independently predicts the presence and angiopraphic extent of stable coronary artery disease, J Int Med, 2008 Jan 16

Amar S, Periodontal disease is associated with brachial artery endothelial dysfunction and systemic inflammation, Arterioscler Thromb Vasc Biol., 2003 Jul 1;23(7):1245-9

Andriankaja OM, Periodontal disease and risk of myocardial infarction: the role of gender and smoking, Eur J Epidemiol, 2007 Sep 8

Arbes SJ, Association between extent of periodontal attachment loss and self-reported history of heart attack, J Dent Res, 1999 78(12);1777-82

Barilli AL, Peirodontal disease in patients with ischemic coronary aterhosclerosis at a University Hospital, Arq Bras Cariol., 2006

Beck J, Periodontal Disease and Cardiovascular Disease, J Periodontol;, 1996; 67:1123-1137

Behle JH, Periodontal infections and atherosclerotic vascular disease: an update., Int Dent J, 2006 Aug 56 (4 Supp) 256-62

Bimstein E;, Serum antibody levels to oral microorganisms in chldren and young adults with relation to the severity of gingival disease., Pediatr Dent;, 1991 Sept;13(5):267-272

Blum A, Periodontal care may improve enodthelial function, Eur J Intern Med, 2007 Jul;18(4):295-8

Bokhari SA, The relationship of periodontal disease to cardiovascular diseases--review of literature., J Pak Med Assoc., 2006 Apr;56(4):177-81

Carroll GC, Dental flossing and its relationship to transient bacteremia., J Periodontol, 1980 Dec; 51(12):691-692

Chong PH, Periodontal disease and atherosclerotic cardiovascular disease: Confounding Effects or epiphenomenon?, Pharmacotherapy, 2000 20(7):805-18

Clothier B, Periodontal disease and pregnancy outcomes: exposure, risk and intervention, Best Pract Res Clin Obstet Gynaecol, 2007 Jun;21(3):451-66

D'Aiuto F, Periodontal infections cause changes in traditional and novel cardiovascular risk factors: results from a randomized controlled clinical trial., Am Heart J., 2006 May;151(5):977-84

D'Aiuto F, Periodontal disease and C-reactive protein-associated cardiovascular risk., J Periodontal Res., 2004 Aug;39(4):236-41

Deliargyris EN, Periodontal disease in patients with acute myocardial infarction: prevalence and contribution to elevated C-reactive protein levels, Am Heart J., 2004 Jun;147(6):1005-9.

DeStefano F;, Dental disease and risk of coronary heart disease and mortality., Br Med J, 1993 March 13;306(6879):688-691

Desvarieux M, Periodontal Microbiota and carotid intima-media thickness: The oral infections and vascular disease epidemiology study (INVEST), Circulation (J Am Heart Assn), 2005 111;576-582

Desvarieux M, Relationship between periodontal disease, tooth loss, and carotid artery plaque: the Oral Infections and Vascular Disease Epidemiology Study (INVEST)., Stroke, 2003 Sep;34(9):2120-5

DiCorleto PE, Participation of the endothelium in the development of the atherosclerotic plaque;, Prog Lipid Res, 1986;25(1-4):365-4

Dumitrescu AL., Influence of periodontal disease on cardiovascular diseases., Rom J Intern Med., 2005;43(1-2):9-21

Elter JR, The effects of periodontal therapy on vascular endothelial function: a pilot trial., Am Heart J., 2006 Jan;151(1):47

Engebretson SP, Radiographic measures of chronic periodontitis and carotid artery plaque., Stroke, 2005 Mar;36(3):561-6

Faria-Almeida R, Clinical and metabolic changes after conventional treatment of type 2 diabetic patients with chronic periodontitis, J Periodontol, 2006 Apr;77(4):591-8

Ford PJ, Cardiovascular and Oral Disease Interactions: What is the Evidence?, Prim Dent Care., 2007 Apr;14(2):59-66

Ford PJ, Inflammation, heat shock proteins and periodontal pathogens in atherosclerosis: an immunohistologic study., Oral Microbiol Immunol. , 2006 Aug;21(4):206-11

Franek E, Chronic periodontitis in hemodialysis patients with chronic kidney disease is associated with elevated serum C-reactive protein concentration and greater intima-media thickness of the carotid artery., J Nephrol., 2006 May-Jun;19(3):346-51

Grau AJ, Recent infection as a risk factor for cerebrovascular ischemia., Stroke, 1995 Mar;26(3):373-379

Grau AJ, Recent bacterial and viral infection is a risk factor for cerebrovascular ischemia: clinical and biochemical studies., Neruology, 1998 jan;50(1):196-203

Grau AJ, Associaiton between acute crebrovascular ischemia and chronic and recurrent infection., Stroke, 1997 Sep;28(9):1724-1729

Grayston JT, Chlamydia pneumoniae- strain TWAR and atherosclerosis., Eur Heart J, 1993 Dec;14 Suppl K:661-71

Grayston JT, Chlamydia pneumoniae (TWAR) in atherosclerosis of the carotid artery., Circulation, 1995 Dec 15; 92(12):3397-3400

Guha N, Oral health and risk of squamous cell carcinoma of the head and neck and esophagus: results of two multicentric case-control studies, Am J Epidemiol., 2007 Nove 15;166(10):1159-73

Guiglia R, Periodontal disease and cardiovascular disease: correlation or simple coincidence?, Recenti Prog Med. [Italian], 2007 Jul-Aug;98(7-8):426-32

Herzberg MC, Effects of oral flora on platelets: possible consequences in cardiovascular disease., J Peiodontol, 1996; 67:1138-1142

Higashi Y, Periodontal infection is associated with endothelial dysfunction in health subjects and hypertensive patients., Hypertension, 2008 Feb;51(2):446-53

Hujoel P, Periodontal disease and coronary heart disease risk, JAMA, 2000 ;284:1406-1410

Hung H, The association between tooth loss and coronary heart disease in men and women, J Pub Health Dent, 2004 Fall;64(4)

Hung H, Oral health and peripheral arterial disease, Circulation (J Am Heart Assn), 2003 107;1152-1157

Hung HC, The Association between tooth loss and coronary heart disease in men and women, J Pub Health Dent, 2004 Vol 64 No. 4 209-15

Jackson LA, Specificity of detection of Chlamydia pneumoniae in cardiovascular atheroma: evaluation of the innocent bystander hypothesis., Am J Pathol, 1997 May; 150(5):1785-1790

Joshipura KJ, Periodontal disease, tooth loss, and incidence of ischemic stroke., Stroke., 2003 Jan;34(1):47-52

Kaisare S, Periodontal disease as a risk factor for acute myocardial infarction., Br Dent J, 2007 Jun 29

Kaisare S, Periodontal disease as a risk factor for acute myocardial infarction., B Dent J, 2007 Aug 11;203(3):E5

Kiechl S, Chronic infections and the risk of carotid atherosclerosis: Prospective results from a large population study, Circulation (J Am Heart Assn), 2001 103;1064-1070

Kiran M, The effect of improved periodontal health on metabolic control in type 2 diabetes mellitus, J Clin Periodontol., 2005 Mar;32(3):266-72

Kuo CC, Detection of Chlamydia pneumoniae in aortic lesions of atherosclerosis by immunocytochemical stain., Arterioscler Thromb, 1993 Oct;13(10):1501-1504

Kuo CC, Chlamydia pneumoniae in coronary arteries of young adults., Proc Natl Acad Sci USA, 1995 Jul 18; 92(15):6911-6914

Kuo CC, Chlamydia pneumoniae (TWAR)., Clin Microbiol Rev, 1995 Oct;8(4):451-461

Kuo CC, Detection of Chlamydia pneumoniae in atherosclerotic plaques in the walls of arteries of lower extremities from patients undergoing bypass operation for arterial obstruction., J Vasc Surg, 1997 Jul;26(1):29-31

Kweider M, Dental disease- fibrinogen and white cell count; links with myocardial infarction?, Scott Med J, 1993 Jun; 38(3):73-74

Laitinen K, Chlamydia pneumoniae infection induces inflammatory changes in the aortas of rabbits, Infect Immun, 1997 Nov; 65(11):4832-5

Lakio L, Pro-atherogenic properties of lipopolysaccharide from the periodontal pathogen Actinobacillus actinomycetemcomitans, J Endotoxin Res., 2006;12(1):57-64.

Larsson B, Cardiovascular disease risk factors and dental caries in adolescents: effect of a preventive program in Northern Sweden, Acta Paediatr, 1997 Jan. 86:63-71

Latronico M, Periodontal disease and coronary hearet disease: an epidemiological and microbiological study., New Microbiol., 2007 Jul;30(3):221-8

Liao W, Endotoxin: Possible roles in initiation and development of atherosclerosis, J Lab Clin Med, 1996;128:452-60

Loesche W, Assessing the Relationship Between Dental Disease and Coronary Heart Disease in Elderly U.S. Veterans, JADA, 1998 Mar 129: 301-311

Loesche WJ, Periodontal disease as a risk factor for heart disease, Compend Contin Educ Dent, 1994- Vol XV- No8 976-92

Lopes-Virella MF, Interactions between bacterial lipopolysaccharides and serum lipoproteins and their possible role in coronary heart disease., Eur Heart J, 1993 Dec;14 Suppl K: 118-124

Lopes-Virella MF, Immunological and microbiological factors in the pathogenesis of atherosclerosis., Clin Immunol Immunopathol, 1985 Dec;37(3): 377-86

Lopes-Virella MF, Atherosclerosisi and autoimmunity, Clin Immunol Immunopathol, 1994 Nov;73(2):155-67

Mager DL, The salivary microbiota as a diagnostic indicator of oral cancer: a descriptive,non-randomized study of cancer-free and oral squamous cell carcinoma subjects., J Tranl Med, 2005 Jun 29,3(1):27

Mason M, Are heart attacks contagious?, Hippocrates, 1997 11(12):42-45 49

Mattila KJ, Dental infections as a risk factor for acute myocardial infarction, Eur Heart J, 1993 Dec; 14 Suppl K: 51-53

Mattila KJ, Viral and bacterial infections in patients with acute myocardial infarction., J Intern Med, 1989 May; 225(5):293-296

Mattila KJ, Association between dental health and acute myocardial infarction., BJM, 1989 March 25 Vol 298:779-81

Mattila KJ, Role of infection as a risk factor for atherosclerosis- myocardial infarction and stroke., Clin Infect Dis, 1998 Mar; 26(3):719-734

Mattila KJ, Dental infections and the risk of new coronary events: prospective study of patients with documented coronary artery disease., Clin Infect Dis, 1995 Mar; 20(3):588-92

Mattila KJ, Dental infections and coronary atherosclerosis., Atherosclerosis, 1993 Nov;103(2):205-211

Mayeux PR, Pathobiology of lipopolysaccharide, J Toxicology Environ Health, 1997 Aug 8;51(5):415-435

Meier CR, Acute respiratory-tract infections and risk of first-time acute myocardial infarction, Lancet, 1998; 351:1467-71

Meskin LH, Focal infection: back with a bang!, JADA, 1998 January Vol 129

Meurman JH, Oral health, atherosclerosis, and cardiovascular disease., Crit Rev Oral Biol Med., 2004 Nov 1;15(6):403-13

Meurman JH, Dental infections and general health, Quintessence International, 1997; 28: 807-811

Michaud DS, A prospective study of periodontal disease and pancreatic cancer in US male health professionals., J Natl Cancer Inst., 2007 Jan 17;99(2): 171-5

Moutsopoulos NM, Low-grade inflammation in chronic infectious diseases: paradigm of periodontal infections, Ann NY Acad Sci, 2006 Nov,1088:251-64

Nieminen MS, Infection and inflammation as risk factors for myocardial infarction, Eur Heart J, 1993 14 12-16

Noack B, Periodontal infections contribute to elevated systemic C-reactive protein level., J Periodontol, 2001 Sep;72(9):1221-7

O'Donnell CJ, Antithrombotic therapy for acute myocardial infarction., J Am Coll Cardiol, 1995 Jun; 25(7 Suppl):23S-29S

Offenbacher S, A perspective on the potential cardioprotective benefits of periodontal therapy., Am Heart J., 2005 Jun;149(6):950-4

Oz SG, Beneficial effects of periodontal treatment on metabolic control of hypercholesterolemia, South Med J., 2007 Jul; 100(7):686-91

Paju S, Is periodontal infection behind the failure of antibiotics to prevent coronary events?, Atherosclerosis, 2007 Jul;193(1):193-5

Paunio K, Missing teeth and ischaemic heart disease in men aged 45-64 years., European Heart Journal, 1993 14 Supplement k- 54-6

Penn MS, Macromolecular transport in the arterial intima: comparison of chronic and acute injuries, Am J Physiol, 1997 Apr;272:H1560-70

Pucar A, Correlation between atherosclerosis and peiodontal putative pathogenic bacterial infections in coronary and internal mammary arteries, J Periodontol, 2007 Apr;78(4):677-82

Pussinen PJ, Endotoxemia, immune response to periodontal pathogens, and systemic inflammation associate with incident cardiovascular disease events, Arterioscler Thromb Vasc Biol., 2007 Jun;27(6):1433-9

Pussinen PJ, Systemic exposure to Porphyromonas gingivalis predicts incident stroke, Atherosclerosis, 2007 Jul;193(1):222-8

Ridker PM, Inflammation- aspirin and the risk of cardiovascular disease in apparently healthy men., N Engl J Med, 1997 Apr 3- 336(14):973-979

Ridker PM, Prospective study of endogenous tissue plasminogen activator and risk of stroke., Lancet, 1994 Apr 16;343(8903):940-943

Ridker PM, The effect of chronic platelet inhibition with low-dose aspirin on atherosclerotic progression and acute thrombosis: clinical evidence from the Physicians' Health Study, Am Heart J, 1991 Dec; 122(6): 1588-1592

Ridker PM, Clinical characteristics of nonfatal myocardial infarction among individuals on prophylactic low-dose aspirin therapy., Circulation, 1991 Aug;84(2):708-711

Rodrigues DC, Effect of non-surgical periodontal therapy on glycemic control in patients with type 2 diabetes mellitus, J Periodontol., 2003 Sept;74(9):1361-7

Rosenquist K, Risk factors in oral and oropharyngeal squamous cell carcinoma: a population-based case-control study in southwestern Sweden., Swed Dent J Suppl., 2005;(179):1-66

Schillinger T, Dental and periodontal status and risk for progression of carotid atherosclerosis: the inflammation and carotid artery risk for atherosclerosis study dental substudy., Stroke., 2006 Sep;37(9):2271-6.

Seinost G, Periodontal treatment improves endothelial dysfunction in patients with severe periodontitis, Am Heart J., 2005 Jun;149(6):1050-4

Seymour GJ, Relationship between periodontal infections and systemic disease., Clin Microbiol Infect., 2007 Oct;13 Suppl 4:3-10

Slavkin H, Does the mouth put the heart at risk?, JADA, 1999 Jan 109-113

Soder B, Risk for the development of atherosclerosis in women with a high level of dental plaque and severe gingival inflammation., Int J Dent Hyg, 2007 Aug;5(3):133-8

Spahr A, Periodontal infections and coronary heart disease: role of periodontal bacteria and importance of total pathogen burden in the Coronary Event and Periodontal Disease (CORODONT) study, Arch Intern Med, 2006 Mar 13;166(5):554-9

Stolzenberg-Solomon R, Tooth loss, pancreatic cancer and Helicobacter pylori, Am J Clin Nutr, 2003; 78:176-81

Syrjanen J, Dental infections in association with cerebral infaction in young and middle-aged men., J Intern Med, 1989 Mar; 225(3): 179-184

Syrjanen J, Infection as a risk factor for cerebral infarction, Eur Heart J, 1993 Dec; 14 Suppl K: 17-19

Syrjanen J, Preceding infection as an important risk factor for ischaemic brain infarction in young and middle aged patients., Br Med J (Clin Res Ed), 1988 Apr 23; 296(6630):1156-1160

Syrjanen J, Vascular diseases and oral infections, J Clin Periodontol, 1990 Aug: 17(7 Pt 2):497-500

Syrjanen J, Association between cerebral infarction and increased serum bacterial antibody levels in young adults., Acta Neurol Scand, 1986 Mar; 73(3):273-278

Tonetti MS, Treatment of periodontitis and endothelial function., N Enjg J Med, 2007 Mar 1;356(9):911-20

Tu YK, Associations between tooth loss and mortality patterns in the Glasgow Alumni Cohort, Heart, 2007 Sept;93(9): 1098-103 Epub 2006 Dec 12

U.S. Dept Health, Periodontal (Gum) Disease. Causes, symptoms and treatments., US Dept Health & Human Services. Natl institue of health. Nathl institute of Dental and Craniofacial Research, nidcr.hih.gov NIH Publication No. 06-1142

Valtonen V, Thrombo-embolic complications in bacteraemic infections., Eur Heart J;, 1993 Dec; 14 Suppl K:20-23

Valtonen VV, Infection as a risk factor for infarction and atherosclerosis, Ann Med, 1991; 23(5):539-43

Velly A, Relationship between dental factors and risk of upper aerodigestive tract cancer, Oral Oncol., 1998 Jul;34(4):248-91

Vilkuna-Rautiainen T, Serum antibody response to periodontal pathogens and herpes simplex virus in relation to classic risk factors of cardiovascular disease, Int J Epidemiol., 2006 Dec;35(6):1486-94. Epub 2006 Sep 22

Wu T, Examination of the relation between periodontal health status and cardiovascular risk factors: serum total and high density lipoprotein cholestero, c-reactive protein, Am J Epidemiol, 2000 Vol 151;3: 273-82

Wu T, Periodontal disease and risk of cerebrovascular disease, Archives of Internal Med, 2000; 160:2749-2755

Zheng TZ, Dentition, oral hygiene, and risk of oral cancer: a case-control study in Beijing, People's Republic of China, Cancer Causes Control., 1990 Nov;1(3):235-41

About the Author

Dr. David Ostreicher is a graduate of Columbia University where he earned his Doctorate of Dental Surgery, Certificate in Orthodontics and Masters in Public Health. He also holds a Masters of Science in Nutrition from the University of Bridgeport, where he served as a professor of nutrition.

Dr. David (as his patients call him) has been a guest on CNN and has been interviewed by Regis Philbin, Barry Farber, Geraldo Rivera and has had dozens of other radio and TV appearances. He has written over 100 articles for scientific and lay publications, and is a lecturer for AlignTech Institute, the continuing education branch of Align Technologies, Inc., the makers of Invisalign®.